We Must Carry On

A True Story of Overcoming Tragedy

BOB THOMAS

Bob Thomas
12/13

Copyright © 2013 Bob Thomas

All rights reserved.

ISBN-10:1492268283
ISBN-13:978-1492268284

DEDICATION

For my angel Samantha watching from above, you are my inspiration and my strength.

To Lori, Noah & Victoria, all that I do is for you. I never imagined that I could one day have a family such as this.
A special thanks to my brother-in-law, Ted for capturing the image in my mind and transferring it to the cover artwork.

CONTENTS

1	An Introduction	Pg #1
2	In The Beginning	Pg #7
3	The Curtain Drops	Pg #21
4	Interlude 1 – Building Your Life-House	Pg #43
5	A Brave New World	Pg #51
6	Samantha	Pg #57
7	The R.O.C.K.	Pg #81
8	Interlude 2 – Your Path	Pg #91
9	Truths Revealed	Pg #97
10	We Must Carry On	Pg #113

1 - AN INTRODUCTION

The following pages have been a long time coming. Memories fade, and I am thankful for that. Repressed memories hide in the merciful fog, until a gentle breeze of clarity cascades down between the mountains of my subconscious, bringing them as clear as a summer morning. I will try to guide you through the patchwork for some semblance of continuity, and apologize for the inconsistencies in my timeline. I've never been a fan of stories with flashbacks, jumping to and fro like a malfunctioning time machine. It's ironic that this memoir, if you can call it that, will not follow a firm timeline that I would prefer. Recollections blur over time, and although I am eternally grateful for that fact, it will leave gaps in my story. I will resist the temptation to fabricate and dramatize to improve the flow, for there is already too much drama and my recollections foggy to the point that some details may be inaccurate. I will try my best to recount the historical aspects as best I can, for it is a history that should not be repeated.

These pages have been delayed for many reasons, although nearly all can be categorized under one basic emotion – fear. I fear that those mentioned in this book will not understand the reasons for it being written. I fear that people will change their view of who I am based on what happened to me. I fear that some people will read these pages and the words will wash away their fog; fog which they depended on to navigate their daily lives. While I believe that the concealment of evil only proliferates its existence; there is a time and a place for sharing, and that time must be your decision. Some things can't be unlearned, sometimes ignorance is bliss; but always knowledge is power.

I have changed the names of the parties involved, to protect their innocence; for they <u>are</u> innocent and that should never be questioned. As I open my heart and share my deepest secrets, I plead for you to ignore that curiosity-filled urge to dig further. One would not need very adept investigative skills to determine some identities, but that has been the over-riding reason for the ongoing stalling of this creation. I have made a conscious decision to accept the consequences of writing this; while they have not and should not be forced to do so. To those parties, I sincerely apologize for any distress, and urge you to put this down if you are not absolutely sure that you are ready to proceed.

Many new authors might encourage their friends and family to read their first manuscript before publication. At least they would become early buyers and potential positive critics of your work. In my case, I almost hope that my relatives and those that I grew up with do not read this. I do not want them to have to relive certain aspects of my past. Putting the past in your rear-view mirror and driving far away is often essential to happiness. I am delving into my past, jumping into that mirror, so that outsiders can understand and learn from it. I hope that readers walk away feeling hopeful, knowing that challenges can be overcome. I do not want pity or sorrow. I certainly do not want those who lived these horrors to have to relive them if they have managed to leave their history behind.

I do not intend to instill a negative attitude before you even reach the end of chapter one, for I am writing this to create hope not despair. There is an old African proverb –"Smooth seas do not make skillful sailors." I can testify to the validity of that belief, for I know I would not be the man I am today without the cyclonic disasters which I have endured. At the same time, those storms nearly broke me on more occasions than I care to admit. Pounding steel in a blacksmith forge to the point of near fracture, in order to create a precision blade, also makes for many ruined blades. I am proud to declare that I survived that forge; the intense heat and the incessant smashing and tearing down of my psyche.

Even as I type that sentence, I don't believe it. Despite my determination to make myself believe that I am a better man, I know that I have dozens of fractures that threaten my resolve each day. Although I have struggled to become a man superior than I thought I could ever be; a damaged, some would say war-torn, psyche still resists the full acceptance of newfound self-confidence. Laughter in a hallway still creates a nagging sensation that the laughter is directed at me. Sometimes I feel unworthy of the love that I have been given and am my own worst critic. On a good day, I can look back at the positive things that I've done and accept them with pride. Most days however, I know I could have done more and would rather give credit to fate. Pride may be the downfall of man, but the lack of it also leads to despair.

Society has come to view depression as a disease, but the degree of infection and the long-term ramifications to the survivors are not recognized fully. Prolonged depression has a permanent impact on your emotional capacities. I feel like a recovering alcoholic, thankful for so many days of sobriety, but always aware of how a single drink could push me back into the abyss.

The best analogy for depression I can concoct is that of a surfer on the ocean of life. The water below his board is the dark murkiness of clinical depression. For most people the current and buoyancy are enough to keep you above the surface. Having positive things around you, such as a loving family, purpose, and sufficient wealth adds to the size of your board. These things provide stability and reduce the chance of falling into the depths below. Everyone dips themselves into the water at some point; this is natural and an unavoidable part of life. We can't appreciate joy without experiencing sadness. We can't truly appreciate life without an awareness of death.

Falling off your board is easy, even for those surfers who seem to be professional. Weather conditions change frequently; maintaining balance during a hurricane nearly impossible. The water near the surface is tepid, allowing you to swim for a while. While you can't maintain the speed through life which you could while on your board, you can still make progress. Days and weeks of swimming without getting back on your board to rest though, will take its toll. Muscles reach the point of exhaustion; cramps halt your progress and you start to sink deeper.

Drowning in this ocean is not as fast as in a real lake or river. Significantly denser than air, it takes more effort to move and you tire easily. Those who know that they have a perfectly sound surfboard inches above them can use that hope to keep swimming just below the surface for weeks, months, even years. If they are lucky, a shift in currents may propel them upwards to grasp that board of life. They may be able to summon up all their strength in one blast upwards and push up to the light. However the easiest way is when another surfer reaches down into the darkness and grabs their arm, hoisting them to safety. You must accept that reaching arm to make it topside.

Eventually your clothes become saturated, weighing you down and dragging you deeper. When the sunlight fades, you reach a depth where no lifeguard or fellow swimmer can reach your outstretched hand. At this point, you can only save yourself. All sense of direction is lost as you tumble through the void. The darkness now feels like home and you can easily forget your former life up top ever existed. The vast emptiness is all-encompassing and you drift aimlessly, waiting for death. The perception that there is no hope of returning to the surface creates a yearning for the end. Death becomes the new goal, rather than surfacing.

You must not give up! You must not surrender to the void of despair and hopelessness. You must reach down into your very core and remember what the warm hope of the sun above felt like. You must believe that the sun does still exist somewhere up there. You must accept that even if your board above seems devoid of loved ones or even the necessities of life. You must believe that you have the power to change things and that good will prevail again. There is a point where you must make a conscious decision to trust your gut as to which way is up and propel yourself back to the surface. Fight with every ounce of strength and reach out to the surface. We will be there to grab your hand and pull you up so you can rest and regain your strength.

It is absolutely imperative that you don't give up. It is hard to remember which way is up, the darkness surrounds you as you float in a sensory deprivation chamber of despair. If you falter, if you forget what the warmth of hope and love feel like, you will sink deeper into the void. The pressure at these depths can crack your very mind. The physical pain from your exhaustive swimming can give way to a complete lack of feeling which seems worse than the pain. You feel nothing, floating aimlessly, unable to connect with anyone. As the pressure builds you can no longer fill your lungs with air. At this point, you will do anything to end the pain. This is last call. This is your last chance. You either end it or try one last-ditch scream for help and hope there is a submarine nearby to rescue you.

Now I ask you, successful surfer, look around as you plod or speed through your day; watch for fellow surfers who may be dangling limbs into the water. Watch for heads bobbing in the water, coming up less frequently as they gasp for air. Watch for empty boards floating aimlessly around you. Call out to them, reach down into that murkiness, for there may be fingers grasping desperately for aid.

I have spent far too much of my life in the water. Treading water until the cold depths below beckoned for me to return. Part of me felt that I did not deserve to float above, in the warmth of the sun. My home was in the darkness below, cold and alone. Any trip to the surface was temporary and undeserved.

It is often a very gradual depression which cycles as the tides ebb and flow. There is often no discernible reason, but that undertow is strong and unforgiving all the same. Sometimes, I kept a couple fingers tethered to my board and recovered quickly. Other times it was harder to maintain my belief that the warmth was just above my fingertips and that I deserved to be back above that surface.

Years ago, I reached the bottom and had become oblivious to the direction of top-side. I had forgotten what the warmth of the sun felt like; my skin pruned from being submerged too long. It wasn't a saviour in a submarine or an epiphany of a newfound potential future that rescued me. To this day, I can't be certain of the cause for my change of heart. I used to think it was cowardice, fear of the choking convulsions as the real lake-water filled my lungs. Now I know that it was divine intervention/subconscious prediction that I was meant to do something in this world. It was over a decade later before I truly realized that undeniable truth.

Looking back, it terrifies me how close I was to squeezing that trigger a little further. How close I was to finding the right cocktail of pills and alcohol. How close I was to losing my footing and slipping beneath the surface on that final brisk morning. How close I was to never reaching this day, being able to see the good that I have done and the amazing legacies which my wife and I have created. I see the promise of hope and joy in their eyes, and am eternally thankful for finding the resolve to fight the darkness.

Life can be hard, life can be downright nightmarish; but if you persevere and find a way to overcome your hardships, life is worthwhile. Loss can be a better motivator than the fear of loss. Hope and love can weather hurricanes, if you believe strongly enough. Every day I am determined not only to avoid being a consequence of my past, but to recycle that pain and transform it into the fuel to make me a better man. This is not a passive task, and I wish that I could say I was successful in this endeavor. Each day I look down and see the murky depths below, and I tremble.

2 - IN THE BEGINNING

I was born in Sarnia, Ontario, a border city with a strong focus on the petro-chemical industry. My parents moved north to a small town in central Ontario when I was six months old. My father, we will call him James, was a carpenter by trade, and built a small cottage near the lake for us to live in. It was a simple structure; assembled quickly, meant only to shelter us while our real house was built up on the hill.

My parents were hard-working folks and Dad always had dreams. His first big idea, which was what sent us northward to begin with, was to build a campground near a lake. They purchased a couple hundred acres with substantial lake-frontage, built our cottage and set to work. I think I was three or four years old when the main house was finished and we moved in. It still wasn't anything fancy, but a big improvement from the green and white three room cottage at the beach.

Roadways were built around the front acreage, a washroom building constructed, and power run for guests with trailers. As the years went by, we focused more on seasonal visitors who left their trailers year-round and spent most weekends at our park. One elderly fellow winterized his trailer and lived year-round on the edge near the woods, away from the noise of the seasonal visitors. I remember that he played an old fiddle and the place always smelled of pipe smoke.

Random guests in tents and popup campers came and went. A small store was built farther down the hill, where Mom sold bread, milk, and candy. We would mix up all the different penny candies and make grab bags for five or ten cents, which the guest children loved.

A couple hundred metres past the back of the actual trailer park, we had a small animal farm. It wasn't a petting zoo type of farm; more of a carryover from my mother's farming background. We had pigs for pork and chickens to provide fresh eggs. A couple times a year, one of the pigs would get free and venture into the trailer park. Most of our regulars can likely still remember seeing my Dad running after a pig, yelling "Sooey, Sooey". He had a crooked old cane carved from a branch, which he used to guide the runaway swine back to their pen.

We had a couple boats moored at the dock, big wooden ones with seats for eight. Dad would take whoever wanted to try their hand at water-skiing. We even had an old aquaplane for those not quite ready for individual skis. Dad taught a lot of kids to swim in our private beach as well, but I never learned. Looking back, it's odd that I couldn't swim when I grew up on a lake and watched my father teach others this basic skill. My sister, whom we will call Leslie, took to it quickly; and would go out on the aquaplane but never ventured to the actual skis.

The trailer park was fairly successful, providing limited but sufficient income for us during the tourist season. As did most of the locals that depended on tourist dollars to survive, we were forced to find other means during the off-season. Dad logged our many acres, providing firewood to those who lived nearby, as well as occasional carpentry work. He built a large log house for a neighbour once, and erected a natural stone fireplace at a friend's cottage. I remember how sore he was after splitting stones all day. Dad was a hard worker, no matter what he was doing.

Mom, we'll call her Jenny, took a job as the secretary at the school where Leslie and I attended. The school was quite small, to match the size of our town. I think we had fifty-four children there, when I attended. There was a kindergarten classroom, one class for grade one and two, another for grade 3 and four, bathrooms, a tiny library and the principal's office. A small desk had been squeezed into the front of the office for my mother to work her half-days.

I was always the smallest boy in class, the youngest to wear glasses, and my asthma kept me from participating in gym class. Schoolwork came easy for me, but the social aspect was a struggle. I had friends though, and except for one incident where I was left hanging on the coat rack at recess, I wasn't bullied much - considering my shy personality and diminutive stature. I think those first five years would have been much harder if I had attended a larger school.

At the end of grade four, everyone at my school had to move to a larger full-size elementary school in a neighbouring town. This school had over three hundred children and was over half an hour bus ride. The bus stop itself was a shared pickup for the four children that lived on the other side of the lake and those on our side. This was a one kilometre walk to the end of our road, then almost another km to the midpoint beside the lake.

My sister switched to the big school two years before me, and she had trouble with the transition. She started getting headaches which we presumed to be from the fluorescent lighting and the crowded halls. A decision was made to allow her to switch to a smaller school that wasn't really in our district but was a comparable distance away. This happened to be a school which our mother now also worked at as part-time secretary. Although none of her friends from elementary grades went to this school, it had just over a hundred children and was a more comfortable environment.

When the time came for me to move on from our tiny schoolhouse, it was an easy decision to go to the same smaller school as my sister. I was still terrified and knew not a soul in my class. I still remember how awkward I felt that first morning. From my viewpoint, everyone was staring at me, pointing and laughing at the little freak. I had to be calmed down in my Mom's office before I could be taken down to be introduced to my new class.

I was the new kid being bussed into a school where nearly everyone else lived within bicycling distance of each other and had been friends since birth. I was, once again, the shortest kid in class including the girls. My permission slip due to asthma that had previously allowed me to stay inside for all gym classes didn't hold as much water here. I had to go out with the class but if we were running laps or doing anything remotely physical, I would end up needing my inhaler and sit by the wall for the duration.

There were no major issues with the other kids; my perceptions that I was ostracized were greatly overdramatized in my mind. Eventually I made friends and the next four years were largely uneventful. I was still at a disadvantage; being a "bus kid" made it impossible to hang out with classmates. We were the very last kids on the bus route; actually past the end of the route. Since we were not really going to the proper school, adjusting the route to include us was not an option. Getting a ride with Mom was limited as she only worked a couple days a week at each school. Most days, Dad would have to drive us to the bus-driver's house so we could start the route with her.

We normally were dropped off before she even came out to start the bus. In the winter we would be shivering on the cold vinyl seats while the old diesel struggled to warm up. On many mornings we could still see our breath and would scratch at the frost on the windows for the first ten to fifteen minutes of the forty-five minute journey.

One thing that has changed dramatically in the past twenty years is the recognition of a "Snow Day". The roads up north are windy and full of hills; not ideal for winter driving to say the least. Our bus driver was determined to get us to school, and it took a lot for her to cancel our trip. This was a decision made by each driver, not someone on the Board of Education watching a weather report over their morning coffee. If the mercury had dropped below minus thirty and the bus wouldn't start, despite the block heater, she'd get a boost. If the roads were bad, she drove slower; sometimes staying in first or second gear for most of the route. "Better late than never" was one of her favourite sayings.

There was one unpaved side-road that we had to go down to pick up two other children that was always the trickiest section on icy or snowy days. Near the beginning of the road was a large hill with a fairly tight corner halfway up it. One day we tried three times to get up that hill before she gave up and went back to the highway; those two kids were getting a snow day. We were all white-knuckled and nervous as she slid back down the hill each time. I wonder now if she would have been so persistent if the bus had been carrying more children.

Classes were still combined and the curriculum scheduled as such; some geography topics were covered in grade seven for some and others in grade eight. It seems odd now, but it allowed for full classroom learning at the time. It also created a larger social group that was separated every other year, but essentially travelled through their elementary education together two years at a time. I was essentially a loner, but with such a small group everyone tends to be somewhat involved.

This bond didn't hold for those of us who lived on the fringe or beyond, and had no choice but to go to their proper high school. I ran into one or two old classmates a couple times after grade eight graduations, but no life-long friends came from that period. For grade nine, I was again destined to be the new kid, as most of the "minor niners" had been attending the school two hundred metres up the road, rather than the one in the neighbouring county.

High school was filled with nervous tension and awkwardness, as it is with all youth to some degree. It wasn't all bad though, and I survived with no permanent scars. I had friends to sit with on the long bus ride home, and was no longer the last stop. I had friends to play cards with at lunch hour and share jokes with in home-room.

I even lucked out with the dreaded cafeteria experience for that first year when I knew practically no-one. I think it was the second or third week when I discovered that they served french fries every other day, my favourite food and which I'll elaborate on later. I remember coming out of the line with my Styrofoam bowl of fries and glancing around the seemingly enormous room, looking for a spot to sit down.

As I walked slowly down the row of tables, this guy stands up and says "Hey, here's a chair, little guy. You can sit with us." I was stunned and a little suspicious. Although this wasn't officially a "jock table", it contained eight large grade eleven and twelve students. To this day, I don't know whose idea it was to try to welcome the obviously nervous newcomer into their lunch group. There was no ulterior motive, hidden agenda or a suggestion from a teacher or a younger sibling to watch out for me. They saved me a seat every day that first year. I ended up being bus seat-mates with the younger brother of the one football player. A football player whom I heard had hung himself a few years ago. Depression and suicide has no social boundaries. Although we had absolutely nothing in common, they realized my discomfort and made a small/huge gesture that was appreciated and made a big difference in my high school experience.

The academics came easy to me, but I struggled socially, never feeling like I belonged or was worthy of friendship. I never dated in high school, even after I had my driver's licence. I obtained my motorcycle licence before my car licence. During grade twelve, I rode a mid-sized cruiser – a black Suzuki 650 Savage. My savings from working at the track, a small loan from my parents and a great deal from a friend at the dealership made that dream come true. I would pass the school buses each morning and again every night. Riding that bike made me feel cool, and special. Despite the opportunity that being a guy with a bike could have offered me socially, nothing changed. Looking back, I think I might have at least had a shot at getting a date if I'd had the courage to ask. That type of courage requires self-confidence, and that was in very short supply.

I was still the small, shy, four-eyed nerd with asthma. Although I always felt inadequate and socially inept, I wasn't really bullied that much in high school. Sure, it happened once in a while, but it wasn't like I spent years in legitimate fear of being beaten up. One winter day, a couple guys picked me up in the hallway and carried me outside. They swung me back and forth between them, gaining enough force with their pendulum swings so I flew pretty high when they heaved me into the snow. Unfortunately, and unbeknownst to them, the freezing rain the night before had left a half-inch of ice on top of the couple feet of snow. The speed and angle which my bare arms and neck broke through that ice made it feel like glass. They thought my scream was from the shock of the cold snow, until they saw the blood. It could have been much worse, but a lesson was learned that day. They regretted their actions long before the principal laid down his punishment. They hadn't meant to harm me, but as is often the case, what starts as a funny prank can lead to serious harm.

After high school, I went to a community college about a hundred kilometres away, taking business administration. My sister and her future fiancé had rented a house in town so I was able to stay with them. It worked out well; he was a long-haul truck-driver so my living there for my first year prevented Leslie from being alone all week. I focused on my education, maintaining my borderline outcast status. Although I had friends at school, I felt disconnected and thought that I didn't fit in.

My second year was short; I dropped out just before the thirty day cut-off so I could get my tuition back. To say that I left school so I could move out west to be with a girl I met through the summer would be misunderstood. Although that is the hard fact of the matter, the reasons behind such a seemingly romantic but foolhardy decision must be explored first.

Now, my friend, we must revert back to an earlier time and review my non-academic upbringing. While my school life was largely uneventful and fairly boring, my home life was unfortunately a little more noteworthy. We tend to focus on the individual trees surrounding us as we grow up, oblivious of the broad workings of the forest. We may think we understand the connections between our individual worlds, but overlook the rotting disease that spreads in the shadows.

A decade after creation, the trailer park began to lose its appeal for my father. He was a builder, and the park had reached its completion. He needed something new to create, and although he didn't ride at the time, he set his mind towards building a motocross racetrack. The trailer park was sold, with the proceeds just covering the mortgage and debts it had incurred. My grandparents had purchased an adjoining section of land years earlier, fifty acres that actually cut a swathe into the centre of our property. The trailer park bordered the lake and was dissected by a dirt road that led into a series of cottages and houses that wrapped around the back of the lake. To the north of the park lay their acreage, mainly a woodlot with a cleared section bordering a sizeable but stagnant pond, alongside which they had set up a mobile home for summer visits. The highway ran alongside the pond to the west, and our property wrapped around the other two sides. In order to travel from the trailer park to the back area where the track was to be built, you had to traverse their property or circle deep into the woods and enter from the rear.

Dad purchased an older John Deere bulldozer and a very beat up dump truck and began building what would eventually be one of the best sand-based motocross tracks in its day. It started out with just a couple jumps built up in the middle of the field, with a couple of local kids on dirt-bikes coming each day to ride. I look back now and the thought plagues me if there was more to that deal of unlimited track time and training. Within a year, the field had been transformed into a mile-long racetrack with table-top jumps, double jumps, tight switch-backs and a huge sweeping berm at one end, leading into a full-throttle straight stretch. The other half of the field was fenced and setup as parking. A salvaged cottage from the old trailer park had been relocated to the new facility and a tower perched on its roof. A small four-bunk travel trailer was positioned at the edge of the fence as our base of operations.

An agreement was made with the only sanctioning body at the time, the CMA or Canadian Motorcycle Association. Within a couple years, we had three or four full-scale races scheduled through the summer, drawing a hundred plus racers and their families from across Ontario. They ranged from six-year-olds on little 50cc automatics to soon-to-be pro's on 125 and 250's as well as a few open class 500's. The races were two day events which normally took at least two to three weeks to prepare for and we never stopped all weekend. As soon as the last bike saw the checkered flag in the last race of day 1, Dad was firing up the tractor to start dragging out the ruts with a huge steel beam and rollers. A Honda water pump was hooked up by the adjoining river so we could water all through the night to keep the dust down.

Motocross provided a fair share of fun and a great deal of work, but only a meager profit. We expanded into other motorsports; all of which were bike related except for an ill-fated attempt at 4X4 racing. The trucks promised a better return but we actually lost money on that endeavour. Our miles of trails and a single trip around the track became a favourite for the semi-infamous Corduroy Enduro race. This was a 300 mile two-day cross –country ride which used our facility as the overnight camping rest-stop one year. We had to enclose the bikes with fencing and provide security to ensure nobody tampered or worked on the bikes overnight.

Our other claim to fame was a huge spectator event that went on for four years – the National Hill-climb Championship. Bikes that had been modified with extended swing-arms, chains on the rear wheels and many that burned nitro fuel tore up our 500 foot hill in mere seconds. Clearing the hill and dumping dirt over the top to make the proper incline took over a year. Our first event drew nearly two thousand spectators but most of the profits were eaten up by marketing costs incurred by our corporate partner. It was a great event, but once again it was not the financial success that we had hoped for.

Between the hill-climb, sanctioned races and daily practice fees, we kept food on the table and the bills were usually paid. The winters were tough though; the purse-strings pulled even tighter. We tried to start a ski resort, but with no accommodations and significant distance from any major population, that venture folded very quickly. This was another business that had potential but without adequate investment capital, our hopes could not be realized. Logging and selling firewood was the only stable source of income to supplement Mom's secretary and subsequent housekeeper income.

At the time, I never really thought that we were "poor". We were never on welfare or on any assistance, but the baby bonus cheques were always eagerly anticipated. Mom taught piano lessons five nights a week, ranging from one to three hours each night. It was much needed income, and she enjoyed it.

Although the plan was to build a large log house on the property owned by my grandparents, the entire time was spent living in the mobile home which they had purchased for future retirement. It was fairly large, as far as mobile homes go. The living room at one end was 10 X 12 with a pop-out on one side that housed our couch perfectly. A narrow hallway ran along the side adjoining the rooms, just wide enough for a single person. The kitchen had a large pass-through to the living room but with the ceiling mounted cupboards and the piano on the other side; you couldn't really pass anything into the living room.

Our air-tight woodstove was located in the kitchen on the hallway side, so you couldn't traverse the entire trailer without navigating around it. That stove put out a lot of heat, but the inadequate insulation kept the bedrooms chilly. Winter mornings usually involved a quick blanket-wrapped dash down the hall to stand close to the piping warm fire.

 Down the hall was my room behind a folding curtain door with a magnetic latch. My room was nearly 8 X 6 with a closet cut in that added much needed extra space. My bed consisted of a thin single mattress suspended on a steel spring bed frame that was supported by the closet frame on one end and a pair of 2x4's on the other. It filled the entire side of the room. A wooden dresser-desk with a fold down top was the only other furniture which filled up the remaining floor-space. A bar-stool finished off the design.

 We had a 12-inch black & white television with a broken channel knob perched on the top of my dresser-desk. We only received 3 channels, each of which required going outside to turn our antennae with a large monkey wrench. Changing the channel on the TV required grasping the small plastic piece, which the missing knob should have attached to, with a pair of need-nose pliers. Despite the challenges involved in watching this small TV, it was our main source of evening entertainment.

 Mom's piano lessons each evening forced us to stay outside or retreat to my room. Leslie was usually out, or doing homework in her bedroom at the end of the hall. Dad & I would lie on my tiny bed and watch T.J. Hooker, Star Trek, and The A-Team. On the nights where Mom was teaching a couple brothers, the student on deck would come down and watch with us. Each Thursday night she taught 3 boys that were dropped off together, so the four of us would sit on my bed, backs against the wall with our feet hanging off the edge.

 Next to my room was the small bathroom, complete with tub/shower, toilet, sink and tiny linen closet. At the very end of the hall was Leslie's bedroom. It was always the coldest room, but it had a real door and was almost comparable in size to the living room. It wasn't as long but she had a double bed and there was room for a full dresser. I would have been envious, but I controlled the evening entertainment - the precious television. I considered myself the winner in that little trade-off.

Handing off the private bedroom to the teenage girl in the household seemed logical for a temporary housing arrangement. Mom slept on the couch and Dad slept on a thin mattress that slid under the couch when not in use. It was not ideal, but gave him easy access to stock up the woodstove through the night when needed.

Some people might have described our little home as cozy. This term implies limited size causing proximity to others resulting in a tight knit family environment. While my actual bedroom may have been the extreme example of cramped togetherness, our trailer was more of a house than a home.

The mobile home was meant to be temporary lodgings while we built the log home that never came to fruition. The basement of our future home was dug and the trees for the initial walls were cut down. Twice those logs ended up being sold off when cash got dangerously low. At one point they had even been de-barked and the preliminary notches cut so they could be piled on top of each other into the basic structure. Ensuring we had enough money for mortgage payments to keep our land always took priority over building a home on that land.

Although our living arrangements were small, we always kept them full. We even renovated our small addition/porch into an extra bedroom so that a neighbour could move in. He was sixteen at the time and having trouble at home. Dad took him under his wing and let him move in. It didn't seem strange, at the time. Later on, after Leslie moved out we had other summer tenants; young boys who were eager to stay at a racetrack for the summer. They earned their keep helping to maintain the property and prepare for the races.

We worked hard and they more than earned their room and board. Just cutting the grass in our huge parking lot was a ten hour job. Some tasks weren't bad, like dragging the track and roadways with a huge steel beam pulled behind our Farm-All tractor. Others were hard labour in a hot field devoid of any shade. Sledge-hammering in wooden stakes on either side of a mile long track, moving hundreds of tires filled with rainwater and mosquitoes, raking and levelling the berms and jumps to ensure a safe race. It seemed the chores never ended.

We would take our breaks in the heat of the day, unless it was a race weekend; then every day was a minimum of 12-14 hours leading up to it. Break time meant ride time. Despite the fact that Dad had never raced, he taught many young boys to ride and to race. There were two cottager boys who had become close family friends. When they agreed to ride as an unofficial team for us, the real training began. We would spend hours practicing how to get that vital hole-shot. Being in the lead when you hit that first corner, with the dust and sand from the other 39 competitors behind you could be crucial to winning.

We didn't have the finances for a proper gate-drop starting mechanism so a 4x4 timber had been dug into the ground at the starting point. When the referee dropped the green flag, forty bikes would fly up the first hundred and fifty feet stretch and funnel into a narrow ninety degree corner to line up for the first jump followed by a high sweeping berm. It was the most dangerous part of each race, but being at the front meant you shouldn't be involved in any pile-up.

My life while we had the track was pretty good. It wasn't easy, but all in all it was fun. I rode; I worked, and had other boys around who became good friends. Girls ... they were an entire aspect overlooked until much later. It didn't matter; I had no chance of having a girlfriend anyway, so I wasn't disappointed in my lack of a normal social life.

My long-term goals in life were to finish high school, go to college for Business Administration and take over the family business. I didn't have unrealistic expectations but my future had some direction and I was content. Overall, life seemed pretty good.

BOB THOMAS

3 - THE CURTAIN DROPS

I remember wondering what was going on when Mom said that we had to go my Aunt's. No reason was given, but it was urgent and we had to go together – just Mom and I though. Leslie had been staying there the last few weeks, and I wondered if maybe she was pregnant. Or maybe something had happened between my Aunt and Uncle who had recently divorced?

There were a few possible reasons, along with some implausible ones, but nothing hinted towards the bombshell that was about to fall. I sat in the armchair, while Mom sat on the couch with Leslie and my Aunt on either side of her. My teeth clenched and an intense cloud of fear began to build as Leslie grasped Mom's hand, tears welling up as she began to speak. "Dad has been sexually abusing me."

I looked down at my stomach, but the twelve-pound sledge that had been hurled at my mid-section was as invisible as it was destructive. My shock and disbelief grew as we were told that he had tried "things" with two of my younger cousins. The room started to swim around me, each statement violently shaking my world like a snow-globe.

I remember feeling intense anger as my sister held my hands and asked if he'd touched me. I knew they didn't believe me, even as I proclaimed my innocence. *I need to clarify that I probably mean ignorance rather than innocence. I know that he was the only guilty one.* I couldn't believe this was happening. There had been no warning signs, no indication that my father was an incestuous pedophile. He was a hard-working family man, a man always willing to help out someone in need, especially kids. The boys who stayed with us over the years – that was just to help them out if they were having trouble at home or just wanted to work at the track over the summer. All the kids were comfortable with him and were thankful for the opportunity to ride bikes. There were times when there were six boys sleeping in the little trailer at the track; it was hot in the summer and everyone slept in just their "tightie-whities" to stay cool. There was nothing out of the ordinary.

It made no sense. The allegations came not only from my sister, but also my male cousin who had spent many summers at our place. If he liked boys, than why hadn't he abused me? This just did not add up; something was seriously screwed up and I was going to find out what was going on. I knew Leslie totally believed that what she was saying was the gospel truth, but people can be wrong without knowing that they are lying. Maybe she had lost her mind and was hallucinating? That didn't explain the collaboration from the other family members who had come forward though.

Later that afternoon, I threatened the very life of my cousin. I swallowed all the confusion, fear and disbelief and boiled them in my soul. The anger rose to the top, ready to be skimmed off and hurled at the closest possible victim. I stormed out of the house and drove my cousin to a parking lot a few blocks away, focusing every ounce of self-control on maintaining my shaky grip on reality.

I told him that while I believed their stories that the abuse was real, I couldn't fully accept the fact that it had been my father. "If this goes forward, and Dad goes to prison, and we lose everything, which will happen when this goes public. If this happens, and I find out years from now that you lied to try and back up my sister when it isn't true. If it wasn't him, and we ruin his life for nothing; if that happens, know that I will kill you. I swear to God, I will fucking kill you." I meant it with every grain of my being.

I had seen stories of misguided accusations that were later recounted. I knew that the damage would be irreparable on every level. My threat was not to dissuade my cousin from telling the truth but rather to ensure that it was indeed truth that would destroy my family.

My threats did not deter him though, and that scenario never came to pass. Dad was charged before we returned home, but released on his own recognizance. He denied any wrong-doing. He didn't understand why these accusations were being made, especially from family. We lived day by day for a while, not really talking about it.

I awoke one morning to the sound of my mother screaming. Tumbling out of bed, sliding the accordion door open; I rushed down the narrow hallway to the bathroom. Dad was curled alongside the toilet, naked and covered in vomit. It was a botched suicide attempt, which somehow surprised us. Mom called an ambulance, and he was rushed to the hospital to have his stomach pumped. The police picked him up at the hospital, took him to jail and placed him on suicide watch.

The only memory I have of his incarceration is my single visit with my grandfather and uncle. He suddenly looked so old and broken in his prison uniform, talking to us quietly through the five round holes in the glass. He apologized for scaring us and proclaimed that the overdose was a mistake. A few days later he was able to convince the doctor or judge or whomever made such decisions, that he shouldn't have tried to kill himself and was no longer a risk to himself. He was released shortly thereafter. I knew later that only part of his statement was true, that trying to end his life "using pills" had been a mistake. A "successful" suicide using over the counter medication requires some knowledge of drugs to obtain a lethal concoction; a knowledge which he did not have. More often than not, your body will fight to survive, even if your mind does not want to, and expel the drugs before permanent damage is done. At least that's what the doctor told me, years later when I was rushed to the hospital, covered in vomit.

I'm not sure when the rumours started to circulate, or how widespread they really were. Nobody that I knew ever confronted me about Dad's crimes, yet the business started to suffer. We only ran one sanctioned race the next summer, which had dismal attendance; less than half of our normal amount of riders showed up. We tried to blame it on the long drive that most serious competitors had to make, but they had done so previously. The writing was on the wall, our track was a family-oriented business and nobody would bring their children to a facility run by a pedophile.

We started logging through the summer, stockpiling cords and cords of wood to sell in the winter. That wouldn't pay the immediate bills, so we contracted ourselves out to a local wood-cutting plant. The logs were trucked in and we were paid a flat fee for each cord that was cut, split and piled. It was hard labor without the profit margin that came from providing the logs ourselves, but it paid some bills for a while.

I remember going with my dad to see a mortgage broker at his cottage on a nearby lake. It was the fanciest cottage I had ever seen. I remember thinking that this fellow was either very good at what he did or very good at ripping people off. Our options had run out, we couldn't make our current mortgage payments. We had to refinance or lose our property.

Although I can't remember the exact amounts, I know that the documents signed that night sealed our fate. The penalties for paying off our current first and second mortgage were too high to completely refinance with a new company. We signed off a third and unbelievably a fourth mortgage at interest rates over eighteen percent. The fourth was a tiny amount, in reality it was the cash to make our next three mortgage payments.

That winter we dropped the price of our firewood, which kept food on the table, but our debt continued to grow. Our high interest mortgage payments were too much to handle. We eventually fell into arrears and the bank foreclosed on our land. Our mobile home was safe as we were actually living on Grandpa's land, but the track and most of our woodlot were gone. That was supposed to be my future, taking over the family business and building it up to the success Dad had always dreamed of. But there was no more family and no interest from riders; that future was dead long before the notices were posted on the gate.

 I stayed with Dad until the end. Leslie had been gone long before that fateful announcement and Mom moved out before he was released from suicide watch at the jail. I still somehow held out hope that he might somehow be innocent; I couldn't leave him all alone. The fact that he had never touched me kept that hope alive. There was no plausible explanation for the accusations unless they were true. I had never seen that monstrous side of him and found it impossible to fully believe the hideous truth.

 Although I never fully accepted that he was a monster, I also knew that my support could also be holding him back from confessing and getting the help that he needed. One evening, a couple of months before he finally ended it, I confronted him with a vengeance. I told him outright that I knew he was guilty and hated what he had done. I still loved him, but he had to admit that he was sick and must ask for professional help or he would go to prison. He hadn't reached the bottom quite yet, and I hoped my abandonment would push him to the breaking point and start the road to recovery. He wasn't a monster, he was mentally ill. I started out calmly but it ended with me yelling and him crying as I left.

 Nothing changed. I had given him the opportunity to confess or explain, but he would not or could not do it. I still don't know which is worse – that he knew the depravity of what he was doing or that he thought it was normal. It always circled back to that fact that I had been left unharmed. He denied any wrong-doing to the very end.

The preliminary hearing date loomed closer. Although we never spoke of it; that was the final deadline that loomed before us. The business was gone, my future plans, our family and friends; everything was tainted or destroyed. How life would go on once Dad was in prison was an unknown. How would I be able to maintain the family home myself? Would Mom move out of her rental house and come back here with me? What would I do with the rest of my life? How much information would come out in the trial? What other dirty secrets would be dragged out into the light of day? What would happen to him? Child molesters don't fare well in prison. Despite everything, I loved him and feared the unknown future, for both of us.

The pounding on the door woke me around 8am. I was a little groggy, and felt like I had just fallen asleep. I remember Dad bringing me a glass of Kool-Aid to wash down my antidepressant pills the night before. I didn't like taking them, but they helped me sleep. He watched me swallow and kissed my forehead goodnight, which seemed a little odd, but emotions were raw as the day grew near.

The officer at the door was nice, and he had brought Mom with him. They brought me into our living room, taking a seat on the beat-up couch perched in the pop-out. Dad had finally succeeded at ending his life. His weapon was our Ford Fairlane station wagon, along with duct tape and a length of our fire hose. He had planned every detail, to minimize the impact on what was left of his family. The only person around to stop him slept soundly, courtesy of two little pills. He drove up to the general store in the middle of the night and slid a sealed envelope under the door, knowing that they would open early in the morning. The note advised the shopkeeper to call the police and send them to our track. He secured the hose, started the engine and wrote his final goodbye letter.

I kept that letter for a long time, but tore it up in a rage a few years ago. That is an excerpt that will not be included in this tale; most days I'm glad that I can't reread it. He went on for two full pages, both proclaiming his innocence and pleading for forgiveness for his sins. He couldn't understand why we were doing this to him, (TO HIM!!!) but he was still proud of us and wished he could have been a better father. He claimed that he was ending it all, not to avoid punishment, but to prevent us from being humiliated in court. The letter didn't really end, but trailed off near the bottom of the second page. His normally poor handwriting became erratic and nearly illegible as the fumes began to overpower him. The police said, the pages were still on a clipboard lying on the seat beside him, the pen on his lap.

In general, I believe suicide is not a reasonable alternative to solve or more accurately avoid a problem. People can change, people can create good things from the blackest depths, and everyone is capable of making the world a better place in their own way. However, his final action was the right thing to do. While it was in part his cowardice and fear of what would happen to him in prison, (his short stint was under the guise of suicide watch and his charges were kept quiet), it did avoid further pain for his victims. More importantly, it eliminated any chance of his eventual freedom and further abuse of more innocent children.

Some would argue that he could have received the "help" he needed and have had his deviant behaviour eradicated. While I firmly believe that people can change and self-improvement is an essential part of humanity, I question the validity of this belief. Often rehabilitation only requires a change in circumstance, environment or improved mental health and well-being. In other situations we must err on the side of caution, for the sake of the potential victims.

At the same time, in a world that cherishes rights and freedoms, the determination of guilt cannot be taken lightly. My father's life was destroyed the moment that he was accused. The inherent uncertainty and often lack of physical evidence in abuse cases makes reasonable doubt a difficult thing to disprove.

It is always and undeniably the rights of the child that must take precedence. Children are the future; protecting them at all costs must always be of paramount importance. Whether my father killed himself to avoid punishment or to protect us from further scrutiny is irrelevant in one regard. His action ultimately protected other children from abuse at his hands.

Does the pedophile suffer from a mental illness that can be cured or is it a genetic predisposition that can only be suppressed rather than removed? While I proclaim that people can change, I also argue against giving someone such an opportunity. Maybe some actions justify the removal of such a second chance. Was my father aware of the harm he was doing or did he think it a normal part of education? These are questions that I cannot answer with complete conviction. Did my father do the right thing by killing himself? Yes. Should he have done it years earlier when he first realized (if he did) that he could not control his evil desires? Yes, without a doubt.

Was he aware of his evil actions? Did he think he was just "educating" his victims? If he thought his actions were "normal", then why had he never touched me? He loved me, but never in that "special" way. So did he not love me enough to show me what physical love was? Or did he love me enough not to? If he was sick, or had been abused himself as a child and thought that it was normal, why was I the only child unmolested? If he knew what he was doing was wrong, then he was truly evil incarnate, fully deserving the worst punishment imaginable.

My untarnished innocence brought much confusion and self-loathing over the years. Thoughts that seem ridiculous when spoken out loud by a rational mind are undeniable in the dark psyche of a tortured young mind. The conscious realization of the guilt I felt only manifested a few years ago in the form of a terrifying repetitive dream.

But I'm getting ahead of myself again; I haven't shared my revelation regarding my own abuse yet. In order to get to that point, we must first journey to the most recent trauma in my life. To understand that fully, we need to explore how I started fresh after my life up north imploded. Before we can reach that point of rebirth, I need to explain my own descent after my father's death.

I was in the midst of summer vacation after my first year of college when I first fell in love. Or so I thought at the time, and in retrospect it bore only the slightest resemblance to such a beautiful emotion. We will call her Sherry.

Sherry lived in Alberta but had come out to spend her summer with her childhood best friend, whom had moved out here years earlier. I had ridden into town to grab some fries at the local restaurant where her friend, we'll call her Donna, worked. Our routine chitchat led to an introduction and somehow ended up with me inviting them both to go to a travelling carnival that night in a neighbouring town.

That evening in my '78 Thunderbird, I began my first intimate relationship. She was in grade eleven and I had just finished my first year of college, so I had the older guy thing going for me, I guess. I also rode a motorcycle which added a bit of danger to my undersized goofy looking persona. We spent a great deal of time together over the next three weeks. We had to rush our relationship along, as she was returning home in late August.

Some days were spent at Donna's house, waiting for her alcoholic father to pass out so we could retire to a bedroom to quietly make out. Things progressed quickly and I convinced a good friend, to let us borrow his family's cottage one night. They only used it on weekends, and there was a key hidden under a rock for unexpected last minute guests.

The night started out nervously enough and far from smooth. The neighbour to their right had stayed for the week so we had to sneak in with no lights or risk being interrupted, possibly by the police. That fear was escalated by the fact that we couldn't find the key-rock in the dark, forcing us to break in through a bedroom window. My buddy had purposefully broken the lock mechanism the previous year to allow easy entrance and exits. The unexpected neighbour proximity made lights ill-advised so we made do with a small flashlight that I luckily had in my T-bird's glove compartment. Hormones eventually won the battle with our mutual shyness, eased by the dim lighting. It was not quick as many such introductions to the world of carnality often are, but I remember the awkwardness.

A couple days later, she flew home and I prepared to return to college. We vowed to maintain our long-distance relationship, and it seemed an easy task when you considered our former social activity, or rather the lack thereof. Her family was very strict and I was her first real boyfriend.

The first month of college was difficult. The certainty that I would not have a family business to take over upon graduation, the uncertainty of Dad's own future, and the fear that others would find out about my pedophile father made concentration a challenge to say the least. Now the promise of being with someone who accepted me as I was, but unable to see her drove me to give up on college, at least temporarily.

I withdrew from college, packed my few belongings and headed west to start a new life. The cliché was just as powerful as I climbed aboard the Greyhound as if it were a stagecoach. In reality I wasn't running to her. There was no promising career or even a job awaiting me. We were far too young, but not so stupid to think that this would be the start of our life together. We were both experiencing strong new emotions that we didn't fully understand and couldn't reason past the illogical absurdity of it all. I was running away from the life that had shattered around me. Those whom I trusted were liars, my future plans in ruin, and my understanding of family was a sham. Alberta held not the promise, but at least the possibility of a new life, and that was enough for me.

Three weeks later, I was flying home. Home isn't the right word, and I refer to it that way for geographical reasons only, rather than a descriptive one. Three weeks alone with my thoughts in a small town motel was too much for me. Sherry was busy with school and friends, and her parents while sympathetic to my plight, were not at all happy to see me. Their little girl's relationship was obviously far too serious if I moved across the country to be with her.

Happiness induced from young love and excitement gave way to despair and my depression returned with a vengeance. Sherry began to fear for my life, and her concerns were not unjustified. Twice I walked down to the train-tracks, filled with uncertainty and a healthy dose of fear. Out here, I had no access to guns or drugs, no lakes or even a tall building or bridge to hurl myself from. The train seemed promising but I feared that I could get thrown and be doomed to life in a vegetative or paralyzed state. My life was bad enough; being trapped in a body with no ability to end it was my greatest fear.

I didn't want to hurt her; she had done nothing to deserve someone as screwed up as I was. I finally came to two conclusions: I needed to go home to confront Dad, and I couldn't continue the emotional torture that I was putting Sherry through. I walked the couple miles across town to the high school dance. I had blown off the invitation a week earlier so I was not expected. I spent fifty dollars of my quickly dwindling and unequivocally sad life savings on a heart pendant for our three month anniversary which was two days away. I gave her the box and told her that it was over. I told her that I had been a fool to come all this way and that I didn't really love her. She wasn't as sad as I anticipated, but I could feel her anger. She already knew our relationship was doomed. I walked back to the hotel in tears and booked my flight home.

I used to wonder sometimes where my life would have led if I had stayed in Alberta. If I hadn't returned to take care of business that I needed to take care of. If I had taken a job in Alberta at the local grocery store as a stock-boy and saved up enough money for an apartment. Would I have made anything of myself? I doubt it. I don't think it was ever a possibility, just a minor detour on the road that is my life. It was a foolish mistake, but one that could only have happened at that stage in my life. One that maybe I needed to make, to realize that if there was someone out there who could be attracted to me, maybe there was someone else. I had thought she was a life preserver cast down for me to grasp, but I had to let go in due time.

I had much swimming left to do, now was not the time to float on the tides. I had not finished the current disastrous chapter of my life, so trying to start another was not a viable option.

The time around Dad's suicide, funeral, and my moving in with Mom is permanently grey. The sequence of events is lost to me. I remember sitting on a concrete barrier in the parking lot of the funeral home, with two friends trying to console me. I didn't know why I wasn't crying. I had shut myself off somehow; an instinctual subconscious distancing of myself from the horror of it all. The ability of the human mind astounds me to this day. Not just the power of reason and logic, but the subtle ability to forget the things that need forgotten in order to survive. It is our ability to turn off an emotion in order to survive a traumatic event. Many people in combat situations likely wouldn't be able to return to the battlefield if they couldn't flip that switch.

The problem with switches is that they can malfunction at inopportune times. Fuses will blow, circuits will short, and sometimes they are flipped back on purposefully. Emotions make us human. Our feelings and how we react to our experiences make us who we are. Without joy, hate, fear, love and ambition, we would be closer to an android regardless of our physical composition. Despite that innate necessity, we all wish sometimes that we couldn't feel. When the pain becomes unbearable, the anger uncontrollable, the despair overwhelming, we yearn to flip that switch. We want to zone out and detach ourselves from whatever is crushing our resolve. That switch, however, is more of a breaker, triggered by an overload and the rating on that fuse is constantly changing. Finding that breaker panel is nearly impossible, hidden in the deepest darkest abyss.

If your breaker blows too many times, or you live in that "turned off" environment for too long, the effects can be nearly permanent. The lights may not just come back on automatically when your surroundings eventually change. Trust me - they will change at some point. Running on such a low wattage makes it hard for others to believe that you still function properly. A spotlight with a corroded contact, loose bulb or spent battery can still function, even if just intermittently. In today's world though, many of us are viewed as faulty and not worth the effort to be refurbished. We are cast aside like so many disposable coloured Mallory flashlights.

Much of my life after Dad's death was spent in a low wattage world. Everything was dim for I could not handle the harsh realities visible in the light. While his life was over, I still had to endure each day. Although I could no longer see a destination ahead, I was still mindlessly moving along the tracks.

Determined not to be another welfare case, I landed a job as a data entry technician at an accounting firm a couple towns over. The gas costs running my Thunderbird back and forth ate up a good portion of my paycheque and the drive in winter threatened my position altogether. I rented a house with two other young guys just a few miles away. I can't for the life of me remember how we got together; we had no mutual friends or history. Regardless, we were only room-mates for about six months or so. One of my room-mates considered himself a ladies man despite having a girlfriend since freshman year of high school. She stayed over most weekends and they would fight like cats and dogs. I avoided most of those disasters by heading "home" for a couple nights.

Mom had rented a small farmhouse across from the lake where I grew up. It was tiny, not just a small old house, but actually tiny. My family, especially on Mom's side were all quite short, and this house was made for us. The kitchen counter was at least eight inches below standard, causing discomfort for any guest who happened to volunteer to help with the dishes. The stairs that led up to the bedrooms were laughably narrow. Carrying anything upstairs required holding it in front or your elbows rubbed the yellowed wallpaper. You couldn't quite call it cozy, but it was close enough for us. She was always glad to see me those weekends, bag of laundry in hand.

I started drinking and partying. My job was tedious and I didn't see any future in it. My employer quickly realized that my heart wasn't in it, and when I started missing too many days, I was let go.

Officially it was due to reduced volumes, but I wasn't exactly the stellar key-puncher they had hoped for. Unemployment and the resulting cheques were just the kick-start I needed to speed up my descent to nowhere. My roommates and I gave up the house rental and went our separate ways, but not without one final keg party in a now furniture-free house. It was nice not worrying about furniture getting broken or drinks being spilled, but with no place to sit down people didn't stick around long.

The only good thing that came out of my time at that house was the beginning of a very dysfunctional relationship. Did I say good thing? That is as far from the truth as you can imagine. However, it brought me to the brink that I needed to reach in order to climb out of my spiral. We will call her Daphne, and she opened my eyes to a world of sex, drugs and alcohol. It was a world that I had been visiting frequently anyway, minus the sex part.

How we met was downright embarrassing, especially for her. My sister and future brother-in-law were having a small party and we had run out of mix. My cousin and I made a run to the convenience store in town, stopping at the liquor store for another bottle of Canadian Club, of course. Cruising back through town, we saw two girls standing on the sidewalk. With my inhibition/inebriation scale tipping quite nicely, we pulled over and invited them to the party. The older girl declined, but surprisingly Daphne accepted and climbed into our car.

A few drinks later, and after some mild groping in the driveway, she hitched a ride home after giving me her phone number. She hadn't made a very good impression on my sister, but I was thoroughly impressed and eager to see her again. Although her phone digits were correct, and the fact that neither of us had much going on in our lives, it still took three weeks to get together again.

She finally called me back and asked for directions to our rental house so she could be dropped off. Apparently she wasn't comfortable enough for me to pick her up at her parent's house. After a quick drink with my roomies, we retired to my bedroom. I was unprepared for this girl's sexual appetite once she started drinking. I'm glad I had the unending stamina of a young man at the time.

It developed into a relationship of sorts, although we never dated in the traditional sense. We never went to a movie, only eating out a couple of times. I brought her to a couple parties but she was uncomfortable with people she didn't know so we rarely stayed long. The only time we spent more than a few hours together was one weekend when she stayed the night at Mom's farmhouse. I had moved into the tiny house by that point and Mom was away for the weekend visiting relatives. We actually cuddled in the morning, spending part of the day curled up together on the couch watching videos on vhs. It was nice, but I think the idea of a relationship that surpassed a merely sexual level scared her a bit. Shortly thereafter our nights of drinking, drugging and banging became less frequent.

I really didn't care what happened to me at that time of my life. That reckless "tomorrow may not come" attitude, combined with a girlfriend who only wanted sex when she was drinking or toking led me down a dangerous path. Looking back, I'm surprised I didn't end up in jail or killed in a car accident. I drove while impaired a lot; a couple bottles of booze along with a 12-pack of mix always nestled in the corner of my trunk. I started getting involved with small-time drugs; selling pills, hash and weed to friends. I was by no means a drug dealer, but I wanted to have stuff on hand to share with Daphne. I found myself spending more and more time with the wrong people.

I remember driving a couple friends to Oshawa to make a buy. We were all very small-time, but this time the guys had been saving up. Some of it came from their pogey or welfare checks along with a couple weeks of working construction under the table. It was a drug buy that I should not have been involved in. I was only the driver; the naïve hopeless driver. We came home with two of the biggest bags of pot I had ever seen. I was supposed to stay at buddy's cottage that night, but was exhausted and felt the need for my own bed. Looking back I wonder if that decision was my own or if my guardian angel had steered me away from danger. The cottage was raided by the police that morning. One of the guys involved with the buy was bragging to a girl that he was trying to pick up at a bar in the city. That girl happened to be an undercover RCMP.

I wasn't heavy into the drug scene. It was all pretty casual and nobody ventured past the "gateway" drugs that we favoured. At least not during the time I was there; I lost track of most of those people when I moved away. Weed, hash, hash oil, amphetamines, and mushrooms were the extent of our illicit drugs. I couldn't handle the mushrooms, they made me gag; but some people found them hilarious.

Before I started with Daphne, I stuck to pills. I loved the energy they gave me. I had never been a smoker, and nobody I knew was into needles of any kind. Pills seemed easy, without the negative side-effects, or so I thought.

One night, I drove a couple friends over to a party in the town where I had attended elementary school. I had taken some 357's before we left but they weren't kicking in as strong as normal, so I popped a couple black beauties as well. I was bouncing around the basement like a crazy man. I had too much energy and couldn't stop shaking. It was like I was vibrating from head to toe; my hair felt like it was standing straight up. I even asked if they had a woodpile that I could go move and re-pile just to burn off some energy.

Actually, there was one time that I tried something harder. I know my guardian angel was watching me that night, arms crossed in disgust but still watching over me. I was feeling particularly reckless that night and a friend had brought acid to the party. My normal group of friends were split on their opinion of the drug. Everyone had heard horror stories about bad trips and semi-humorous ones of the stupid things that they had done while under its influence. None of us would ever shoot up or snort anything, so acid was pretty much the limit. Its appearance in our social circle was pretty rare and I have to admit that I was curious.

My buddy, we'll call him John, who owned the cottage that we were partying at, had tried it before. We both "dropped" around seven pm. I was accustomed to the fairly quick impact of my "bennies" and was unsure if anything was happening. Then I noticed that the dartboard on the wall was becoming cartoon-like; it was shifting into a weird hyper-coloured swirling orb. My good friend, we will call her Jessie, squeezed my hand gently when she saw me tense up with a hint of fear as I sat there silently. "I think it's kicking in" I whispered to her softly.

Some guys from another town showed up, uninvited and unwelcome. There was some bad blood between one of our guys and one of theirs. Something along the lines that a girl told him that she was single, while her boyfriend had a different opinion. John had a stupid catch-phrase that he used whenever he was high —"I'll bite your big toe right off." Although I don't recall hearing him say it that night, the idea was lodged in my screwed up subconscious. One of the uninvited guests had his leg crossed and was dangling his sandal-clad foot annoyingly close to John's face. I didn't see him bite it off, but I noticed that John was chewing his gum with his mouth open. Everyone seemed oblivious to the loud smacking noises, but I couldn't turn away. My eyes widened as I saw a bloody fat toe rolling back and forth in John's mouth. It seemed like forever before I had the inclination that this could just be a hallucination from the LSD.

I turned to Jessie to share this odd little tidbit, but she had turned away from me, ignoring my persistent tugging on her shoulder. I called out to her repeatedly but to no avail. My irritation changed to horror as I looked down to see a glowing ember fall from her cigarette onto John's puppy. He had curled up in the little dog bed beside the couch, unaware of the ashes being flicked onto his adorable little head. The ember appeared more massive than any cigarette could produce, but it fell right onto his paw. I jumped from my seat and tried to swat the smoldering cinder from his paw. My hands became ghostly in consistency and I flailed pointlessly. I yelled at Jessie, "You're burning the dog!"

"What are you talking about? We sent the puppy to John's parents for the night. Like half an hour ago."

I looked down at the empty dog bed in disbelief. At this point I realized that I could not trust anything that I saw. I thought that I was in a safe environment, that my friends would take care of me in this vulnerable state. Jessie was keeping an eye on me, but in my mind there were so many crazy things happening while she kept ignoring my pleas for help. She told me the next day that I spent most of the night staring blankly and only spoke a couple times, despite my vivid memory of conversations that went on for hours.

At one point Jessie asked Darryl to take us for a drive, thinking the cold winter air would do me good. The roads were icy and we slid all over the road. I looked out the side window, expecting to see snow-banks, but instead was greeted by flames. We were driving alongside a ledge that dropped straight down without a single guardrail to be seen. Flames shot up, spewing lava into the dark night skies; we were on the edge of Hell. I remember Jessie complaining that I was squeezing her hand too tight; apparently she was unaware of the eternal flames flashing up beneath our tires.

Suddenly, we plowed head-on into another truck. The other driver had come out of nowhere. He must have been driving without any headlights; another stupid game that we played while drinking. Racing back from a party we would pass each other with our headlights off, the road illuminated only by moonlight. None of us were hurt, but Darryl was furious. He grabbed the tire iron from behind the seat and leaped out of his truck to confront the other driver. Darryl started yelling profanities, ordering him out of the other truck. It was another blue 4x4, surprisingly similar to Darryl's own GMC. My eyed widened as Darryl climbed out of the headlight-less truck and started to apologize to the ranting Darryl. I honestly thought that angry Darryl was going to beat the living tar out of apologetic Darryl. He always had a temper and his submissive alter-ego seemed to be pushing him past the brink. Angry Daryl pushed Apologetic Darryl against the grill of the second truck and returned to us. There was no major damage so we headed back to the party.

The party was pretty much over when we got back. Eventually I could look at things for more than a minute without them changing into some twisted cartoon version of themselves. Darryl gave me a ride home, without a single hellish flame in view. I was so glad that trip was over, but the ripples carried on through the next morning. The blankets rippled with serpents swimming beneath the sheets as I tried to sleep.

I swore I would never do acid again, and never did. I was terrified by my inability to differentiate between reality and fantasy. That decision was reinforced by a story that I heard much later regarding that very night. Apparently while we were on our 4x4 ride through Hell, John became paranoid that someone was planning on stealing his stash. He came out of the bedroom with a shotgun, warning them it was time to move on. He was disarmed and talked down; everything was civilized and somber when we returned.

Some dangerous situations were avoided out of pure luck, it seems. Looking back, I'm astounded that I survived those years despite the continued reckless behaviour and my own inability to care if I lived until the next dawn. Driving under the influence and dangerous driving on unforgiving roads was the norm. These were stupid things that could have taken my life, or the life of an innocent. That is the part that makes me hate the person I was at that time. Although I always tried to help a friend in distress, I risked their very lives every time I got behind the wheel. The fact that I could have paralyzed or killed other young people scares me now, but I was ignorant to that logic during the time.

Other dangerous situations that could/should have prematurely ended my life were intentional. Depression ebbed and flowed constantly, both before and after Dad's death. They were not cries for help; most attempts were done in private and never spoken of. Although I held firm to my belief that I had not been abused, the knowledge that my father was a monster ate away at me every day. My future had been taken away; my past was all a lie. My low self-esteem hindered my ability to build a new meaningful life. I didn't expect to live to my twentieth birthday, and I am astounded to this day that I have made it this far.

At one point, I bought a package of razor blades and drove to a local motel. I didn't want Mom to be the one to find me, so I needed a safe location to end it. Although it was off-season for tourists, I was unaware of the hefty cost of a room for the night. The fact that I was twenty dollars short was the only thing that stopped me that night. By morning I had come to my senses and went back to my dreary life.

Another day, I had been crying most of the morning, to the point of exhaustion. I just wanted it over. I couldn't handle the pain any longer. I scribbled a note, "Don't come in. Call the police. I'm sorry." I taped the note on the door at Mom's rented farmhouse, locked and chained the door. I loaded Dad's old Winchester rifle, which I had inherited. That had been a sure sign that nobody had a clue regarding how messed up I really was. Firearms and depression do not go well together. I sat on the couch with the stock of the gun squeezed between my knees and wrapped my mouth around the cold metal. I sat there, sobbing with my thumb on the trigger for what seemed like forever. I'm thankful now for my cowardice that day; for that's what I thought it was, at the time. I realize now that it wasn't weakness but strength that kept me alive. Despite my intentions, I was not quite ready to give up. There was a small glimmer of hope that flickered enough in the black void to make my subconscious wonder if life could indeed be better someday.

One such attempt did not remain a secret, and I should have known better. Dad's overdose attempt had failed miserably and put him in jail on suicide watch, but I thought I could make a better pharmaceutical cocktail. Mom was visiting her sister for the weekend, so I had overnight privacy to finish it once and for all. I wrote another note, which I securely taped to the door. I avoided the inclusion of alcohol to wash down the pills fearing I might vomit before the pills put me to sleep permanently. Anti-nauseates, sleeping pills and painkillers were washed down with Kool-Aid.

My concoction was as ineffective as my father's had been. I awoke at some point and threw up repeatedly before passing out again. The sun was already up when I awoke to hear a scream at the door. I had neglected to remove the note from the door. Leslie was banging on the door as I stumbled to the living room. I tried to assure her that it was a stupid mistake and I was fine, but the level of my depression was no longer a secret. She rushed me to the hospital where they surprisingly did not pump the remains from my stomach. Apparently my vitals were strong and anything that I had not already hurled up would have been in my bloodstream already. I was thankful for being spared that little treatment.

I had to agree to see a psychologist, which continued for a few weeks. Expressing my fears and confusion may have helped a bit at the time. I cleaned up my act for a time and tried to find a job, but nothing dramatically changed.

I can't recall how long it was before my life-changing suicide attempt, when I reached rock bottom and lost track of the direction to the surface. Daphne had moved on, and I was certain that I was unworthy of anyone else's affection. I was destined to be alone for the rest of what I was certain to be a short life anyway. I had nothing to live for and was tired of living.

I wrote a short letter and sealed it an envelope, placing it on the passenger seat of my car. I kept the letter brief; I was determined not to chicken out this time and didn't want to become too emotional while pouring out my apologies. It was early morning with a hint of fog rising above the lake. I had parked across the road from the boat launch beach, the spot from which we would lower our boats into the lake when we owned the trailer park. I left my shoes and socks by the car and gingerly walked down to the water. It was chilly, sending goose bumps up my legs. The water was shallow for quite a distance out before dropping off. My inability to swim combined with no will to live made this a definitive method from which I wouldn't be able to stop at the brink. I misjudged the distance to the drop-off though and stood there shivering. The water level was just below my nose, my lips submerged. I just needed to take a few more steps or plunge forward to let the water fill my lungs. The pain would be over. I would be free of this nightmarish world.

    I don't know why I turned around. I suddenly had an inclination to give life one more chance; not that this crummy life deserved it. Not that I deserved a good life, as unlikely as that was to manifest itself. Regardless, I turned back. I threw my soaking wet clothes into the trunk, donned a pair of shorts I had in the back, and drove home.

    Within a week, I had made arrangements to live with my Aunt and Uncle in Sarnia. I packed up my few belongings and headed south. There was no promise of a better life, but it couldn't be any worse. Maybe I just needed a change in scenery, a new outlook on life. If it didn't work out, they at least had tall buildings to jump from – I couldn't chicken out of that. I can't say that I was filled with hope, but I had nothing to lose. It was worth a shot, one final shot.

4 - INTERLUDE - BUILDING YOUR LIFE-HOUSE

Mankind are creators by our very nature. We are here to build. Some of us build houses, bridges, cars and computers. Others create movies, write songs or even books. We are here to build relationships, make families and procreate to maintain our species. We are here to make the world a better place. In order to do that, we must make ourselves into better people.

There is no "ideal" and there is no perfection. Strive to be a better version of who you were yesterday. Realistic expectations and constant improvement are essential to become the person you want to be.

At the end of the day, take five minutes and review your actions throughout the day. Are you ashamed of what you did today? Did you do anything better today than you did yesterday? Did you have a positive impact on other people? Did you do your best, even if that may have been insufficient in your own eyes or in those of others? Did you have moments of joy? What did you do today that you are proud of?

At the beginning of the day, set small goals that will make today a little better than yesterday. Make a concerted effort to reach those goals. Do the things that you wish you had done yesterday. Don't repeat those things that you regret. Make that positive impact, or make a larger one, or more of them. Think of that person whose opinion you value the most, and ensure that they would be proud of something you do today. It doesn't matter if they see it or are aware of your accomplishment; what matters is that you know.

Day by day, bit by bit, you can build yourself into the person you want to be. It isn't easy, and every construction is different. There are unexpected pitfalls and delays, making the final completion seem like a pipe dream. Not that completion is ever really reached, but you get my point, I hope. We are constantly evolving, but reaching that point where we are justifiably proud of whom we have become – that is the goal.

Think of your life as a house, a custom-built house where you are the carpenter, electrician, plumber and decorator. Family is the foundation upon which your "life –house" is built. Your father is the concrete, and your mother the wooden forms that mold the shape, size and depth of that foundation. Without the union of those two ingredients laying the groundwork for the building of a new life, you wouldn't exist. Grandparents, aunts and uncles are steel rebar carefully laid throughout that foundation, adding strength and rigidity.

In some cases, your early "life-house" needs to be physically moved from that foundation at birth or early in life without any consent on your part. There are foundations out there, many of excellent quality, which are unable to secure contracts for a proper build, and they need to adopt a new structure to customize and build as their own. These secondary locations can become as integral in the creation of your world as the biological foundation that brought you into this world.

In an ideal world, the foundation that supports you during your growth to adulthood is solid and steady. It nurtures and protects you from shifting ground and floods. It provides stability and strength, allowing you to build yourself into the best that you can be. It allows you to design and decorate yourself in different styles; as it is only through trial and error that we find what works best.

Whether the foundation consciously promotes the concept or not, many houses feel that they must look like those around them. They think that conformity and cookie-cutter design will ensure security and stability. The neighbouring houses appear happy and confidant, at least from the outside. Therein lays the problem, my friends. Things are often not as they seem. Rotten timbers may be supporting that roof; the slightest stress or shift could cause the entire building to collapse. Faulty wiring could result in electrocution or a short circuit at an inopportune time.

Even if the structural integrity is sound, neighbours rarely know the depravity and sorrow hidden behind those curtains. The grass may be greener on the other side of the fence but that may not really be due to proper diligent care. That appearance may be the result of carefully placed and balanced manure, or it could a complete illusion – AstroTurf laid to conceal the truth. It is easy to become dissatisfied with your own house when you constantly see or think you see better houses all around you. In reality however, your house is what you make it. You can focus on the exterior only and impress your neighbours or work on the inside. We don't live in our yards; building comfort and security inside is what matters.

As we grow, we start to have more control, more input over how we furnish and design our individual worlds. Our parents will guide us, possibly even restricting the stores that we shop at, but eventually we live in a house of our own making. Guests may leave items behind or the relationship itself can leave a huge impact on the interior design. They can have structural changes that flow through the very architecture of the building and shake your very foundation.

Guests who stay for a while usually leave some trace, although it may be something that you don't even notice. That vase on the shelf that you forget is there or the box of clothes stashed in the attic.

While I hate making generalizations, it seems that "most" people have a need to conform, to fit in, rather than stand out in the crowd. They try to make their house look identical to that on the left and the right. Can you imagine the monotony if we were all the same. There is nothing wrong with being different, being unique, being one of a kind. Standing out is how you gain attention, and how can you make a difference if nobody notices you? So be yourself, express yourself, design and decorate yourself as you truly are. If everyone had the courage to do so, what a beautiful and diverse world we would live in.

Some of us have trouble building our life-houses for we find ourselves in rough neighbourhoods or on uneven ground. Rather than surrounding ourselves with those who would help install some flooring or wire a ceiling fan, we spend our time with those that would vandalize our new siding and stomp on the freshly potted plants. It is a tricky but rewarding feat to build that beautiful house on the edge of a cliff. It is even more rewarding and more worthwhile to help that neighbour shore up his foundation to keep his house from sliding down the ravine.

I equate the different phases of our lives as different rooms in our "life-house." As we progress through our own personal evolution, we not only change the interior design of our house, but also switch to different primary living areas. While you may move furniture from one room to another, you certainly are not the same person with the same interests and traits ten or twenty years earlier.

Unlike physical lodgings, our life-houses overlap with those who are important to us. The living room of your spouse may become so interwoven with your own that it is hard to differentiate between the two. Every action and every item in this shared room impacts both parties, but the electrical and plumbing behind the walls still operate independently and react differently to stimulus.

In the wealthiest of neighbourhoods, people concern themselves with the well-being of their co-habitants and neighbours, rather than just their own house. When I say wealthiest, I am referring to true wealth rather than financial wealth. Although monetary needs are necessary, and lack thereof has a trickledown effect that negatively impacts all other areas, it is not paramount for success. Financial wealth is a vehicle to help transport you where you need to go, rather than the destination. This is an important lesson in your self-evolution.

Consider if you will, a man living in the country twenty miles from the nearest town. If he had a car he could work in town, socialize with more people in town, explore the countryside and have more options in general. However, without a car, he can still live a healthy happy life. He may have to grow much of his own food, and only walk into town once a month for supplies. He will learn the importance of material goods or the lack there-of. He will focus on self-sufficiency rather than how to be a part of the industrial machine. Maybe he will build a cart to attach to his horse and make his own vehicle. Maybe he will become so successful in his own right that the townspeople will come to him.

The point is that real wealth is measured in personal happiness and the positive impact you have on the world around you, not the amount of money in your bank account. Who do you think of when I say "role model" or "personal hero"? Most people jump to famous people who made a difference in the world. Mother Theresa, Ghandi, Martin Luther King, Abraham Lincoln. Others think of more local hero's – firemen, policemen or the minister who runs a food bank down the street. Consider the fictitious superheroes – Superman, Wonder Woman, and Spiderman. All of these people, real or not, are labelled heroes because they help people, not because they are rich.

In many cases, the recognition of their success is heightened because they overcame their own lack of wealth or realize that helping others is more important than helping their own wallet.

When it comes to your own shared house, that focus on other's satisfaction must be balanced with your own happiness. Some people fall into the supportive role too deeply and forget to include their own contentment into the equation. If you devote 100% of your efforts to making others happy, you can become unhappy yourself.

Consider a simple relationship between two partners, without children; their focus to build their shared "house" and strengthen their bond until it is ready to expand into a family. If both parties work in a symbiotic relationship, each strengthening the others weakness, nurturing and promoting both self-growth and their partner's, they will flourish. If each strives to put their partner's needs above their own, both will find satisfaction. However, if one party takes on the support role with no reciprocation, their own needs will not be fed.

Eventually that one-sided devotion will take its toll. It may be unappreciated or just naturally end, leaving that supporter alone with an empty room. Traditionally this would have described the loyal housewife who perhaps gave up a career to raise a family and maintain the family home while the husband advances his own life. In today's world, that paradigm is still common-place but the number of non-traditional scenarios is growing. Regardless of your personal situation, I stress the word balance in everything. Focus on others; for it is by helping others that we grow ourselves. Leave the world a better place than you found out, by whatever means possible. Take the time to make yourself happy as well.

Let's circle back to the house analogy. You spend varying amounts of time living in each room, and you share that room with different people. They come and they go, and some will move with you to the next room or chapter of your life. For some people, this house is a duplex or triplex, for others an apartment building. You can't fully move into a new room until it is the proper time. Some transitions are very gradual, to the point you don't even notice that you moved until that moment of reflection. You may have a recreation room and a living room on the go. As the weeks pass, you find yourself watching movies in the living room since it is closer to the kitchen. You move the sound system into that room since that is where the Blu-ray player is now. One day you realize that you have a fully functional rec room in the basement that you haven't even vacuumed in six months.

Sometimes you need to close the door behind you to eliminate the temptation to go back to familiar digs, and sometimes the people left behind will slam that door behind you. If you're lucky each move will be better than the last, or at least be different enough to allow you to grow into the person that you were meant to be.

Sometimes the room burns down around you while you sleep, or becomes infected with termites that gradually eat away at the very walls. When this happens, you can try the fire extinguisher or call in the pest control company, but sometimes you need to vacate. You need to believe that there is something for you outside that door, another place to live, another couch to rest your weary head. If you don't step through that doorway, as ominous and unknown as it is, you may risk becoming ashes yourself.

Build your house strong, furnish it with love and don't be afraid to let in guests. The most beautiful houses deserve to be shared. Their design concepts can be taken home with those guests so they can improve their own lodgings. Don't be afraid of change. Change means to evolve, and to evolve is to make better.

Although I say you need to build your house strong, it must be flexible. Earthquake prone areas often have houses built of bamboo rather than concrete or hard woods. Their elastic properties allow flexibility so they don't crack or crumble under stress. Strength does not necessarily equal rigidity. The importance of knowing when to be firm and when to be flexible cannot be overemphasized.

There is one more aspect of this analogy that I'd like to share, before we return to my story. Everyone has a safe hidden in their house somewhere. In this vault we hide our deepest darkest secrets, our fears and our nightmares. The primary safe is secured to keep these negative energies from wandering around our life-house, tainting and destroying as it goes. These black gems tend to scare away visitors who could have become permanent guests if they hadn't seen your little horror show so early. Allowing a glimpse into your vault can actually help solidify a relationship at the right time, but the guest must be confidant that you control the vault. They need an opportunity to take an inventory and be convinced that your house is structurally sound enough to consider staying, even for a short time.

Sometimes we put a secondary lock-box inside that safe for the real nasty stuff. These are the things that we won't admit we even have in the house. Sometimes they are memories that get locked away to maintain our sanity. Opening this box sometimes requires professional guidance, for the nightmares inside may awaken and refuse to be put back in the box. Sometimes, it is better to leave the key hidden away forever. In my introduction I noted that some parties mentioned in this book may not be ready to open this particular chest of evil. I hope that this book does not manifest into a key for their personal vaults, for they do not belong to me and I have no right to open them.

My inner vault was shaken ajar in a terrible earthquake a decade ago. I don't know if it was the over-stuffing of the outer safe that caused the breach. Regardless of the identity of the trigger that unleashed the nightmares that had been buried since childhood, a key was unintentionally turned in that lock.

One mental health professional that I dealt with commented, "To be frank, I am surprised that you are able to stand at all." I took his opinion as a word of praise rather than of pity. Now that I start pouring out the reason for my determined survival, I realize why (although how is still a mystery) I was able to continue breathing. My house had to weather these challenges so I could tell you that even the deepest cracks and the strongest hurricanes can be overcome. With strength of will, you can be rebuilt. A house may be blown from its foundation, it may be split in half and fall into the abyss, it may burn to the ground. With strength of will, you can rebuild yourself. You can rise up from the ashes and begin again. When your house is destroyed, you can build a bigger, better house that you can be proud to call home.

5 - A BRAVE NEW WORLD

It was early autumn when I walked through that door into a new level of my life-house. I had tried to leave as much of my former belongings as possible downstairs; wanting desperately to start fresh. I locked the door behind me and disabled the elevator to eliminate any temptation to return. Such a move was of no real consequence; such actions are easily undone and a discarded mental key has a way of reappearing in your pocket at the slightest beckoning. As time went by, I started noticing items that I thought had been left behind had suddenly appeared in my new digs. Some baggage is harder to get rid of than others.

My relatives welcomed me into their real house and I quickly considered it home. I registered for the spring semester at the local college to finish my accounting degree. Many of my cousin's friends became my friends, and I made more at school. Although dating was rare, I was content with my new life. I took a couple part-time jobs at the college to supplement my student loan funds. One job was only three to four hours a week, cleaning the cafeteria after classes while the other involved updating WHMIS files in the school database. Both were tedious and mind-numbing, but despite not paying rent I still needed some income.

The first year and a half was relatively uneventful. I focused on school and spent most Friday and Saturday nights at local bars with friends. We would show up early to get a good buzz going with cheap drinks before the prices went up. Unless the band was really good we rarely closed the place, but spent more than our share of hours nursing our drinks at our table. I started smoking briefly but it was just something to keep my hands busy while waiting for more people to show up at the bar. I never smoked outside of the bar and only had two or three each night. My brief foray into the smokers' realm lasted less than a month. Previously the only time I bought cigarettes was for tobacco to roll with our hash or hash oil in my former life.

My world was changed forever one night by a simple prank call. My cousin had dated my future wife Lori for a very brief period, years earlier in high school. She and a friend had called our house to harass him a bit and I answered the phone. I was much more confidant on the phone than in person, and we ended up hitting it off. We talked for hours and were soon seriously dating.

I was three years older, rode a motorcycle and had long enough hair to tie in a ponytail when riding. She was set to graduate high school in a couple months while I was already in college. That fall she started at the University in Windsor, also studying Accounting. Aside from both of us being inherently shy and our fields of study, we didn't seem to have much in common. Neither of us had really furnished our individual life-houses and we grew together.

After her first year of University, she transferred to Lambton College. Being away from home and from me was harder than anticipated, despite regular weekend visits. She quickly discovered that she did not want to pursue a professional accounting designation, so college would likely be a better stepping stone towards a book-keeping type of job.

A friend who worked for a customs broker at the border found me a part-time job working weekends while I finished school. Upon graduation, I could not find anything accounting related locally, so I accepted a full-time position with the same company.

Twenty years later, I am still in that same industry, although at a much higher level on the corporate ladder.

Lori graduated college one year after me, and we were married that same day. We rented a 2 bedroom townhouse and began our life together. She quickly found work in the accounting department at a local marina while I worked at the border. For a brief period we both worked days, but most of our first five years together were spent with her on days while I worked 4pm-midnights.

After a year of throwing our money away in rent, we purchased our first real home – a small 3-level split in Corunna a couple blocks away from her parents. It had a nice sunroom and a reasonable sized backyard for our dog. Life was pretty good.

In the spring of 1998, we were blessed with our first child – a perfect baby boy whom we named Noah. Two months into Lori's maternity leave, she was offered an accounting job at a fabrication company two miles up the road. It was more money, a two minute drive and would eliminate the time gap between our shifts once she returned to work. Although it cut her leave short, we had to accept.

For the next two years, we were ships who passed in the night. She rose at 6a.m. and left for work at ten to seven each day, returning at 3:30. I passed Noah to her at the door and began my twenty-five minute journey to the bridge for my four to midnight shifts. We were both tired but we were able to avoid daycare and each had lots of time with our young son. We had no idea at the time that this was just the warm-up for our future.

In the fall of 1999, we were informed that we would likely need a bigger house. Lori was pregnant with twins! We knew it was a possibility as Lori's mother was a twin, but it still came as a shock. We were both excited and nervous. Noah's early years had been exhausting with both of us working full-time; how could we handle two babies at once? Neither of us made enough to allow the other to stay home to raise our three children until they reached school age. Regardless, we were in better financial shape than I had been growing up, and we had a strong support network of family on both sides. We knew we would make it somehow, and eagerly awaited their arrival. We also moved to a much larger two-storey house that backed onto a park before the girls joined our clan.

As the days grew longer in the spring, so did my wife's bulging pregnant stomach. The girls were eager to see the world. Lori's water broke in the evening, five and a half weeks before her due date.

Labour was quick, within two hours of leaving the house I became a father to twin daughters. My first beautiful daughter, Victoria, came into the world without issue. I was overcome with joy. Less than ten minutes later, that joy turned to terror when I saw my second baby girl arrive limp and seeming lifeless. My first grey hairs appeared that night. There had been a twin transfusion of blood during the births and I feared my Samantha had passed before taking her first breath.

The doctor rushed her into an ante-room, leaving us unaware of what was going on. Agonizing seconds later a cry emanated from that room, and I wept. Sammy was ok. She was kept in an incubator for a few hours, but that night Lori was able to hold both girls. Despite being five weeks early, they were a healthy weight and we went home a week later.

The girls were pretty good sleepers, so we were not too sleep-deprived once they passed the three hour feeding routine. We bottle fed, one with each girl. Diapers and formula were the highest grocery cost for quite a while; the rate at which they recycled their food kept us hopping.

I was working the 4pm to midnight shift at the office and she arranged to work 7:30-3:30. The extent that we saw each other through the week included a two minute hand-off at the door between our shifts and an occasional mumble through the night regarding which child was crying. We took turns getting up with them through the night, alternating who had to rock which child back to sleep.

Through the week, we were both like single parents. Simple tasks like getting time for a shower became an ordeal. Nap time was a highlight of the day, even if that private time was used to shovel the driveway. Many days, I looked forward to going to work so that I could sit down and rest a bit.

Don't get me wrong, I enjoyed that quality time with my kids. Noah was a great big brother, showing the girls his picture books and always entertaining them. They would dance around the living room until they fell over; exhausting themselves before nap time. I didn't realize at the time how much I would eventually treasure those memories. That's the problem with mankind; we don't realize how important some things are until they are gone. We take family for granted, presuming they will always be there. We rush through life; eagerly waiting for tomorrow instead of enjoying each moment of today.

I didn't fully realize it at the time, but I was living the dream. I was living in a nice house, bigger than anything I ever envisioned owning. I had a beautiful wife that loved me and three great kids that I spent eight hours a day with each and every day. We had a reliable car and I rode a new sport-bike. We were both making a decent wage, with no significant debt outside of our mortgage. Life was good. It was far better than I expected, better than what I felt I deserved. My life had turned around, but I still felt something was missing. Despite my success, I couldn't fully accept my happiness for I still felt that I didn't deserve it.

That sense of unworthiness is hard for most people to understand. The gradual erosion of self-esteem and self-worth has a life-long debilitating impact. The statement "I don't deserve to be happy" seems ridiculous when spoken out loud, but overcoming that subconscious belief is not easy. It's the invisible scars that are the most difficult to treat and that take the longest to heal.

I had random anger issues that I couldn't explain. Some of the luggage that I had brought from my past and stored at the back of my deepest closet would fall off the shelf and tumble out into my den. I pushed them back into the dark recesses and tried to ignore their occasional intrusions into my happy life. I was good at keeping secrets and wouldn't let anyone see my rage. I released it on the highway on my bike, occasionally reliving the high-speed reckless behaviour of my youth. Riding calmed me, bringing me back to centre. I rode to work every day that I could as well as riding for pleasure whenever possible. I had escaped my past, my despair and anguish tucked away in boxes in the back bedroom of my mind. Most days I forgot it was back there; I was cruising now, enjoying a life I had never expected to see.

6 - SAMANTHA

In August 2002, we took a family vacation up north for a week, staying with my mother and her new husband. They had a nice house on a lake a few miles from the town where I had attended middle school. We took the kids out for boat rides and they played in the sand at the edge of the water. We came home a couple days early as Sammy had developed a bit of a cold. It wasn't anything major, but the weather had turned cool and damp so coming home a little early wasn't a big loss.

Sammy's "cold" got worse in the next few days; she began to wheeze in her crib and didn't have her normal energy through the day. Finally, one morning Lori decided enough was enough and took her to the emergency room. We had no idea that our world was about to be turned upside down.

Her chest x-ray was first read as early pneumonia, which seemed bad enough for our little girl. A second doctor looked at the x-ray, luckily, and expressed his concern that it didn't look right. I received a phone call to drop Noah and Victoria at my Aunt's house as we had been ordered to take Sammy to London for further tests. We were scared but had no clue how scared we should have been.

Later that afternoon we were informed that our twenty-eight month old daughter had cancer, specifically Acute Lymphoblastic Lymphoma. She had a tumour the size of a grapefruit in her tiny chest that had nearly collapsed one lung and was pressing on her trachea. Her breathing issue when she lay on one side was due to lack of air as she compressed her one good lung. We were told that the tumour would have grown to its current size in two to three weeks and that if we hadn't come in when we did, she likely would have died in her crib.

Our perfect little world came crashing down around us. Fear, confusion, anger, and denial washed over us; smashing every positive emotion with unimaginable force. Children don't get cancer. Older people get cancer, smokers get cancer, coal-miners get cancer, but not 2 year old infants. This couldn't be real; we were having a nightmare from which we couldn't wake.

Samantha was admitted to begin chemotherapy immediately. This form of cancer was rare for a female child of her age. We were told what they believed was not the cause of her illness, but they had no idea what triggered the illness. It was not a familial illness; for that we were extremely thankful as Victoria had identical DNA. She would have to undergo an intense round of chemotherapy to shrink the tumour before it caused any permanent damage to her organs or resulted in organ failure. They kept us hopeful that she could recover and live a normal life, while maintaining the severity of the current situation.

I wracked my brain trying to figure out what could possibly have caused my baby's illness. The fact that she had an identical twin exposed to the same environment with identical genetic material who was not afflicted puzzled me. We were so thankful for that grace, and engrained a new life philosophy for me. As unbelievably horrible and heart-wrenching as her diagnosis was, it could have been worse. Victoria and Noah were still healthy. I use that phrase frequently, whether it be for a small inconvenience such as a heavy snowfall or a personal illness – "It could be worse."

No matter how bad things are, no matter how many things go wrong at the same time, there is always the possibility that it could be worse. An illness could be impacting other loved ones as well;

physical pain can always be worse. Even if that pain is so severe that you pass out, that loss of consciousness can be a relief. Watching your children suffer causes your own pain, and losing a child is the ultimate gut-wrenching loss. However, being thankful for the health of your other children is essential to carry on. Finding that balance between devoting all your time to a child in hospital without ignoring the siblings at home is a delicate balance that challenges every parent with a seriously ill child.

Our lives had been changed forever; my depression frantically grabbing at my heels, trying to yank me down to the depths again. There was no time for such selfish introverted focus however. I had to be strong for my daughter, my wife and our other two children at home. Months later when things turned from bad to worse, being needed by them was the only thing that kept me alive.

Lori moved into the hospital with Sammy. One advantage, if such a word can be used in such a situation, of having such a young child in hospital was the allowance for a parent to sleep in her room. I drove the hundred kilometres back and forth most days, taking care of Noah and Vicky. Lori's parents and my mother helped immensely during the entire ordeal. I continued working for the first few months to ensure mortgage payments and the like were kept current.

During the initial treatment, I moved into our decent sized hospital room with Lori and Sam on weekends. A rollaway bed in the corner provided reasonable comfort and the necessary proximity which we wouldn't give up.

I brought Noah and Victoria down one Saturday to visit. They didn't understand why their sister couldn't come home and missed her terribly. Watching the three of them sit on Sammy's bed, sharing fries and Mcnuggets is one of my fondest memories of that time. A photo of that meal was my screen-saver for a number of years. They played for a while and then curled up together to watch Barney videos. Sammy tired easily and we had to balance activity with adequate rest.

I remember the first time that Lori noticed that Sam's hair was beginning to fall out as she gently brushed it. Then her little girl locks were gone; there was no longer a quick hesitation to be sure which of my beautiful twin girls I was looking at. Her bald head only made her more beautiful though, something I didn't think possible. I have treasured photos of Noah and Vicky kissing her bald head.

There was a time when I could sing every Barney song and predict every line on many of her videos. I was surprised the VHS tapes didn't burn through with the constant rewinding over and over again. Later on, when we moved to Sick Kids Hospital in Toronto, she started liking The Wiggles as well. I found them annoying much faster than the friendly purple dinosaur, but we watched them continually as it made her happy.

When your child is sick, potentially terminally ill, you do whatever it takes to make them happy. A smile, a giggle, a semi-lying down little dance are valuable gems that you continually mine for. The unrelenting reality looms all around, blacking out the glimmering threads of hope that you cling to in order to wake the next day. Those precious moments of laughter are beaming rays of sunlight that cut through the darkness like razors and fill your heart with joy.

That sparkle in her eye was almost always there, and that alone kept us going. Her treatments were terrible; the vomiting, diarrhea, the endless needles and tests were as cruel as they were necessary. She never let them break her spirit though. The nurses always commented on how brave and happy she always was. They weren't just saying that for our benefit; she was well-known on the floor as an amazing little girl.

As all patients do, she had her good days and bad days. I try to remember the good ones. I wish I'd taken more video of her, but bringing out the camera often brought out the angry face. "Don't take my picture" she'd say. Then softly, "take my blankie" and I'd zoom in on one of her many blankets that my mother had sewn for her. One day I did get a great video of her throwing confetti. She was wearing her pink Blue's Clues pajamas and standing on her bed. When asked what she was doing, she replied simply "throwing".

"Are you making a mess?" I asked good-naturedly.

"No," she snapped with a slight grimace, followed by a big smile. "I'm having a party."

Later that day she realized that the tube that dangled between the port in her chest and her faithful IV pole/companion resembled a skipping rope which demanded to be twirled. Our supplies were limited, but her creativity never was. We made dolls from play-dough, using the plastic needle covers for solid arms and legs. She played doctor with her Beanie Baby cats, taking their temperature and checking their blood pressure.

Beads were another big way to pass the time together. We could have given every patient in the hospital a bead-necklace but we never tied them off. Once the string was full, the beads were slid back into a bucket and then the sorting would begin. The largest collection had come in a tray with twenty different compartments for each colour. Sammy loved to make Lori and I sort them over and over.

Those beads were the regular plastic ones that could be purchased anywhere. Sammy had another collection though; a collection with meaning. These were ceramic "Bravery Beads; each with a significant meaning: pokes, chemo, tests, very bad days, surgeries and transfusions. We have seven necklaces stashed away, reminders of her ordeal and of why we must carry on.

On bad days, we stuck to watching videos to keep her lying down. That was by far how the bulk of our time was spent. She would be engrossed in the make-believe world, often only partially aware of her surroundings. Nurses would take her blood pressure while her eyes never left the suspended television. Distraction is often as essential as nutrition to survive the day.

I still had my work for an occasional distraction during her time in London. We were in the wind-down stage of a two year pilot project that had consumed many extra hours before her diagnosis.

All of the stress and urgency that seemed paramount before that dreadful day suddenly became a trivial means of temporary escape. My heart never left London, but work gave me a change of scenery – a luxury that Lori never enjoyed.

Our health and that of our loved ones is taken for granted, until it is challenged in some way. Then we suddenly realize what really matters and what is just getting in the way. Work is a necessity and that is an undeniable truth of existence. Even those who cast off the industrial nine-to-five existence and live in a commune cut off from society still must work. The soil needs turned, gardens need harvested, livestock need fed, and these activities are all work. Those people may not view it as work, but that is a just their perception. The hired hands at a local farm making minimum wage to pick tomatoes certainly consider it work.

My point is that in today's society, our job tends to define us to a much greater degree than it should. How do you respond when someone asks you, "What do you do?"

"I'm a manager at a retail store." Or "I'm a school-teacher."

The real answer should be "I'm a father, who earns money to buy food and pay my mortgage by supervising others who sell clothes." The teacher's real answer should be, "I try to teach children how to learn new things and instill moral values, which pays my bills so I can feed and clothe my own children."

While neither of these replies would be technically incorrect, the emphasis on the former pushes us further into forgetting what is truly important. The unemployed man feels he has no purpose; the lack of a career or even a job equates to a lack of identity. Many people strive for careers that they deem to be worthwhile, those that directly relate to a positive impact on society. Doctors and nurses are the prime example of this honourable association between earning a living and living for a purpose. Based on my experience I believe that the majority of people choose these fields to help others rather than merely to earn a living. The success in financial terms is a by-product, rather than the underlying reason for the career path.

While these "healers" have a daily and direct impact on the well-being of others, it in no way diminishes the value of the farmer who grows the fruit we consume, or tends the chickens or cattle. The world has evolved far past the point where essential careers are limited to providing sustenance, shelter and healthcare. Specialization and geographic diversity have made the world the wondrous place that it is. Thousands of different jobs have been born out of the complex tapestry that is our industrialized world.

Each person now has a multitude of career choices to select from and the option to change paths is never completely gone. Regardless of your chosen path, it doesn't necessarily define who you are. I work as an office manager to pay my bills but I no longer define myself in that manner.

My primary role is a father and a conduit to help others. I am here to make my children the best they can be and to support them the best that I can. I am here to pass on the lessons learned through hardships I have endured, so others can avoid them. I am here to raise funds for childhood cancer research and awareness for child abuse. That is my purpose and that is who I am, regardless of what corporate name is on my paycheque.

Most days I enjoy my chosen career, and the satisfaction granted from a job well done should never be dismissed. Whether it is something of substance that will endure, or an improved process to create a new corporate efficiency, or a simple monthly report; the completion of the work has merit. However, in the greater scheme of things, changing jobs would not inherently change who you are, at your core.

Who you really are can be changed without a career change, or even without having one. Many people wander through life, wondering what they should be doing. They have an unending yearning to know "Why am I here?" They don't realize that the simplest, most basic reason for being can be enough. Procreation and the subsequent raising of children that believe in the betterment of society can be the most vital job.

My wife and I had a harsh "life-job" change thrust upon us with Sammy's diagnosis. All the trivial day to day issues were sidelined. Our sole purpose was to keep Sammy happy and healthy as long as we could. At that age, we didn't have the option to try and squeeze in much life experience in her remaining months. All she wanted and all we wanted was to spend time together – playing, making bead necklaces and laying together watching Barney.

While we always focused on the good days, the days that she was strong enough to sit up in bed, we had our share of scares.

Life in the hospital was like living on a roller coaster with no safety bar or straps. Looking forward with sunlight and blue sky filling your vision, you feel exhilarated and hopeful while squeezing the hand of your seat-mate. Then the bottom drops out and you plummet downwards. Your heart stops for a brief moment, allowing your mind to contemplate the imminence of the end for that endless instant. Suddenly you corkscrew left and seem to be heading back up on stable ground. Darkness envelops you as you glide into a pitch black tunnel of uncertainty and you lose all sense of direction.

A time comes when you realize that despite all your efforts, all your pleas for help to the onlookers that you race past are for naught. The doctors manning the control tower are flipping switches and pulling levers as if they are in control. If they could only find the right sequence to power down the speed and hit the huge red POWER button that was somehow concealing itself on the massive control panel.

For all their degrees and training, their control over your coaster is flimsy at best. They try their best, but they are only levers and buttons as well in this great mechanism. The engineer is the only one in control, only he can safely disarm the runaway ride. You pray to him daily, pleading and begging for the ride to end. You offer to jump off the ride into the abyss, if only he would activate the safety bar for your child. You scream out at him in rage for allowing such a ride to exist in the first place. He was the one who hit that green button that started this ominous journey. There had been no warning signs, no ticket purchased or gated line to join. We were randomly snatched from the real world and thrown into this nightmare.

The why and the how are over-ridden by the overpowering question of how to make it stop. What will it take to take our baby home and return to our unappreciated healthy lives? You live one day at a time, scared to plan for a future that is so uncertain. Hope is an evil trap that you clutch at wildly, knowing that its' slippery slithering will not allow a firm grasp. You know how hard it will be when that hope is dashed away again, but you can't give up hope for that is all you have left.

At one point in her London treatment, she was given a particularly nasty drug whose effects were intolerable for her tiny body. I received the call late in the afternoon at my office that she was going downhill fast and I had to be there. Luckily I had ridden my motorcycle that day, and at that time my steed was a newer model Honda 600cc sport-bike. It was a crotch-rocket by very definition and I needed its acceleration and superior handling that afternoon. A trip that would normally take over an hour was done in thirty-five minutes, door-to-door. I choked back my tears and focused on maintaining the fine line between maximum speeds and ensuring I made it there in one piece. Traffic was light and I travelled at over 160 kph for most of the way. The last few miles from the highway off-ramp to the hospital were the slowest and most dangerous as I weaved through traffic. Not a single police car crossed my path and while I'm sure I would have secured a proper escort, I didn't want to waste time explaining my need for speed.

Sammy was resting on death's door when I arrived. One of our "regular" nurses left the room in tears, a sure sign of her dire state. It was not her time though, and she made it through the night.

We had many more months on this hellish ride, and many more treasured days to spend with our beloved Samantha. That drop had terrified us and drove home the uncertainty of it all. Hugs became tighter as we prayed that we could keep our baby with us.

Our prayers were finally answered. Sammy's tumour had shrunk and her numbers were stable so she could return home with us. She had to go back for clinic regularly but we had our baby home again at last. Hope seemed to have solidified and allowed a tether to be secured to it, we prayed for good.

I have a brief video of Noah and my adorable twin girls playing in the leaves that autumn with Lori raking them into piles to be jumped in. Sammy's legs were too weak for jumping but she would stiffly bend over and pick up handfuls to throw in the air while Vicky dove into the piles and giggled. This was another fond moment that I treasure as a crown jewel in my collection.

We went to the animal farm together, played on the slides, fed the geese and the baby goats. We were a family together again, suddenly overwhelmed with appreciation for the little things. Our life had returned to relative normalcy and we embraced the miracle that had been provided. The misplaced anger and terror were quickly pushed to the back of our minds, but never forgotten, as we prepared to move forward from the atrocity that we had escaped.

Those days seemed to fly by, and I couldn't tell you how long this reprieve lasted. It came to a jarring end though, despite our thankful prayers. Sammy's scan showed her tumour had returned and was growing again at an alarming rate. The nightmare was far from over, and any appreciation for that interlude was hard to fathom at the time.

We thought that the news of her diagnosis had been hard to stomach, but the return was even harder. Her initial diagnosis had been tempered with positive odds, but after living through her treatment and perceived recovery to have it dashed away was like smashing a bone that had just started to mend.

A second round of chemo was needed to stop its growth. It would be stronger than the first one, an unfathomable punishment in our eyes. She needed a bone marrow transplant at Sick Kids Hospital in Toronto after the treatment. This last round would not only kill the tumour but her own bone marrow - in order to replace it with a new immune system. It was her only chance at survival.

Sammy was re-admitted before the snow began. The tumour reacted well to the new treatment. A major fear had been that it had become resistant from the initial barrage and would not be reined in by chemo alone. The final phase of her chemotherapy which would prepare her for the transplant in Toronto was set for early January. We were also told that transplants are risky and without guarantee. While the odds of it "taking" were high, complications were not uncommon.

As the end of December approached, there was some debate over how to handle Christmas. Our eventual decision was one which I am eternally thankful for. Sammy's health was fairly stable but her immune system was still very much compromised. We could stay in hospital to play it safe; coming into contact with the most innocent of bacteria or common virus could have devastating effects on her treatment. There was a chance this could be our last chance to take her home for a few days; this could be our baby's last Christmas. Those thoughts were never spoken out loud, but the fear was undeniable. I tried to take as much video as I could, and I wish now I had owned a better camera. As grainy as some of those shots were, they are treasured.

We kept the Christmas small as far as visits, fearing that a small illness could wreak havoc on our plans for the transplant. Sammy did surprisingly well, being home seemed to regenerate her. She played with her brother and sister, rarely letting her weakened legs slow her down. There was much laughter and childish giggling in our house that Christmas. It remains one of my fondest memories.

After Christmas we made our first trip to Toronto to see the Children's Hospital. It was an impressive and yet terrifying building. Once her final treatment in London was complete she would be transferred here to the transplant ward. The protocols in place to ensure no germs entered the immune-compromised section seemed very thorough. The recovery ward was equipped with negative pressure so no airborne bacteria could enter. Visitors other than parents could only come to a lobby area outside of the main ward. This would be the middle ground for others to come and check on us.

We were all tested for marrow matches, a crucial fork in the road to a transplant. Luckily both Noah and Victoria were perfect matches. We were surprised to hear that Noah would make a better candidate than Victoria, her twin sister with identical DNA. The doctors explained to us that essentially the transplant would make the new genetic material attack the cancerous cells in Sammy's body as her body accepted the new marrow. If we introduced identical material, her body might not recognize the difference; they were too similar. Noah's marrow however was a perfect match but not genetically identical. The other strange thing that we had not realized in advance was that post-transplant, Samantha & Victoria would be physically identical in looks but Sammy's blood and marrow would now contain Noah's DNA rather than being identical to Vicky's.

Sammy's final chemotherapy treatment in Toronto sole purpose was to completely destroy her immune system, in preparation for the new marrow. It was extremely harsh on her little body but she was a trooper. Her strength and resilience never ceased to amaze me.

The first week Lori was able to stay on a built-in couch in the corner of her room while I made nightly trips across the street to a dormitory style building to sleep. It was a 10 X 10 room with a cot, small dresser and tiny fridge, but was all I needed. A week later our room at Ronald McDonald House became available. I can't say enough how beneficial this was, and highly recommend supporting this charity. Although we rarely made use of the kitchen or other common areas, having a comfortable bed at no cost during our four months in Toronto was invaluable. Due to her young age, we rarely left Sammy alone.

Immediately following the actual transplant, Sammy was in an isolation room where we could not stay the night with her. The measures in place to ensure no contagion could approach the zero-immunity children inside were impressive. Our fingers were raw from the incessant surgical scrubs required before entering the isolation zone. A simple thing like touching your face while inside, required exiting and washing again. We finally obtained permission to bring in a couple of Sammy's stuffed animals which she loved so much. If they fell on the floor, which they often did, they would be taken back to the House to be laundered and returned in a sealed zip-lock bag.

The transplant itself went well. I was very proud of my son that day. He overcame his substantial and justifiable fear to go under the knife for his sister. I could see the inner battle between love and fear in his eyes, but love overcame, as it so often does. He recovered very quickly, to the point where it was difficult to keep him in the bed while we waiting for his release. The five small round scars across his hip bones eventually faded completely. Sammy's numbers slowly climbed and she was moved back up to the transplant recovery ward. It was a ward in that it was a secure section of the hospital with limited access and strict contagion controls. Each patient had their own room and most doors usually left closed. Although we spent many nights at Ronald McDonald House, her hospital room was our primary residence for those four months.

It took a long time to start to forget the words to her favourite Barney movies. I don't just mean the songs either. We watched some of those VHS tapes literally hundreds of times. "Again, Again" Sammy would exclaim once the credits started to roll. They made her happy, and aside from reading to her or stringing beads, we didn't have much else to occupy the time. Eventually she started watching the Wiggles and Veggie Tales as well. Personally I could only handle the Wiggles in small doses, but her dancing and singing along with those animated vegetables always made us smile.

We didn't really bond too much with most of the other parents. Everyone was focused on their own child, and listening to each other's nightmarish tales only made it worse. Cocooning seemed to be a coping strategy for many of us. Aside from brief encounters in the semi-secure waiting area, there wasn't much opportunity for social interaction.

There was one family there who also came from the Sarnia area. Their son, Peter, was 17. His donor had only been a 4 out of 6 match and his graft vs. host disease reaction was very severe. It was a fairly common reaction as the new marrow perceives the host's body as foreign and tries to kill the healthy cells along with the diseased ones. Ideally you want that biological warfare inside the recipient to be graft (donated) vs. tumour, rather than graft vs. host.

His pain was very severe near the end as his new marrow essentially rejected his body. Peter and Sammy had somehow bonded, despite never having met. Peter had made a cat for Sammy from clay a couple weeks before he started his downward spiral, and Sammy reciprocated with a sticker collage card when she heard that he was in pain down the hall.

Another young boy, Johnny, I recall from our time at Sick Kids was someone whom I never actually saw but who had a lasting impact. Some of the patients had small whiteboards mounted on their doors, indicating their name or brief messages. This particular young man, I think he was around eleven or twelve, had boldly proclaimed, "I will beat this, I am a survivor." This simple statement made me smile when I noticed it while walking up the hall to my own little survivor.

A couple weeks later, I noticed his name had been moved to PICCU on the big board by the nurse's station. This board was a basic tool for the nurses to keep track of who was in their section that day. The grid showed each patient's first name, and where they were that day: W (Ward/in own room), TW (transplant ward), or PICCU (Pediatric Intensive Critical Care Unit). The normal pattern for a new arrival was W, followed by TW, back to W and then ideally wiped from the board as they are released. Sometimes patients would end up in PICCU and then come back up to W. Sometimes they went to PICCU and then were wiped from the board. Everyone knew what that meant.

I didn't review the board each day, and was unaware of how long he had been gone. Looking back, his door had been closed and the room dark for at least a few days. That morning, walking up the hall, I realized that his door was wide open. Maybe he was back? I glanced quickly in, only to see his father rapidly stuffing colouring books and stuffed animals into big black garbage bags. I only caught a glimpse of his face, but I knew he had been crying. Despite his valiant determination and positive words on his door, another battle had been lost that morning.

This type of occurrence was not uncommon and steadily fuelled our fear of the critical care unit. Sammy was doing well though, and we kept a strong grip on our hope that we would return home together.

Another terrifying scare crossed our paths that spring – SARS (Severe Acute Respiratory Syndrome). Although there had been no cases in our hospital, we were on lockdown. Visitors were not allowed in the hospital at all for a couple weeks during the height of the panic. Due to her young age and the life-threatening severity, we were permitted entry but only one of us at a time.

Entry to the hospital required not only answering a few health questions, but also temperature checks at the front door. Although the number of people in the hospital was dramatically reduced, we timed our entries to avoid the line-ups. I couldn't enter until Lori had left, so our transition time left Sammy completely alone. Depending on her mood at the time, leaving before the replacement entered her room was often an ordeal.

Lori and I took turns; splitting up the days between being with Sammy and resting back at the House. While it gave each of us some much needed down time, it still added to our over-all stress level.

The basic thin masks that we normally wore when in the isolation room post-transplant were deemed insufficient with such a threat present. We had to wear a much more effective duck-style mask that fit much tighter to the face and had a built in filter, similar to some painter masks. These masks were not designed for long-term use and we usually had severe headaches within an hour of wearing them.

Aside from the actual transplant ward with their isolation rooms; our section was considered the safest place to be. Exposure to the outside world was very limited; the entire area had positive airflow so no contaminants could enter when a door was opened. Everyone knew the fatal consequences that even a common contagion would have, so no shortcuts were even considered.

I remember one day we had to go down to another floor for her cat-scan. Sammy had to wear her little teddy-bear mask and the sheets were pulled up over her head while being rolled down the hallways. Sammy insisted I come with her under the "tent" and the nurse allowed this minor non-compliance. We pretended there were monsters outside, trying to restrain our giggles so they wouldn't hear us. Every little distraction helped to keep the mood light and our thoughts away from the real risks involved.

Outside of the hospital most people seemed oblivious to the potential threat. Watching the media from inside, one might have expected a greater impact on the streets close to the downtown hospitals. Inside everyone was on high alert, but from our standpoint, everyone else was going on with their daily business. The only thing we were concerned with was keeping our child free from any additional threats and getting her home again.

Sammy continued to slowly improve as winter began to finally end. I have video of her playing excitedly in her bed, sit-dancing along with the Veggie-Tales and playing with her stuffed cats. She had a small doctor kit and we would take their blood pressure and listen to their hearts while her nurses did the real thing.

Everything seemed to be looking up. I even went home twice for the weekend to see our other children. On one of those trips, I bought matching birthday presents for the girls. Their birthday was May 21, and we had high but not totally unrealistic hopes that our girls would be under the same roof again by then. I put the two pink birthday bicycles, complete with training wheels of course, in the garage. Teaching them to ride would be a highlight of the upcoming summer.

My mother had moved down to our house to take care of Noah and Victoria while we were gone. They only made it down to Sick Kids once to visit that spring. It was a short visit, but they were all so happy to see each other. I don't know how we would have managed if we hadn't had all that family support.

It was the last week of April, 2003 when our roller coaster crested the top and everything below fell away. Sammy's oxygen saturation levels began to drop. She was put on oxygen and taken down to PICCU – the place we feared the most. The cause was unknown, but Sammy had developed RSV – Respiratory Syncytial Virus. For healthy children it would have been no more threatening than a common cold, but for Sammy, it was our worst fear realized.

Our first trip down to that floor only lasted a couple days; her levels stabilized but had to be kept on oxygen in our room. Sammy didn't like having the big rubber mask on, but thought the hose connected to the wall was funny. It was her elephant trunk and she adapted to this new appendage quite well. Her singing and sit-dancing was now limited to a few moments at a time. She tired very quickly and started to lose the little appetite that she had started to regain.

The doctors tried various treatments but every time they tried to reduce her supplemental oxygen, her O2 sats would drop. We tried not to let Sammy see how scared we were; we had to keep our happy faces on for her sake. She caught me one day though. We were watching Barney together; well actually I was watching her watching the movie. I started to think about what might lie ahead, about how grave the situation really was. This was a dangerous activity when trying to keep an air of hope in this environment. She saw my tears. My daughter, not even three years of age, says to me, "No leaky eyes, Daddy, they won't help."

This piece of advice from such a young child blew me away. Ironically it brings a tear to my eye every time I recall her thoughtful attempt at soothing my sorrow. It is the basis for a line in the song that I would write years later and Victoria would bravely sing at our 2013 Childhood Cancer fundraiser. "Oh my baby, every day, I still try."

There was another tidbit that Sammy shared near the end of her short life. I thought it whimsical at the time, and didn't think twice for any real meaning behind her words until a few weeks later. I had just arrived in her room one morning. The first thing she says to me is, "I can fly Daddy. You can't, you're too big. But I can."

It's strange that the one who was sick, the one who was just a baby, was the one who gave us strength to endure this ordeal. She never lost her spirit; she never worried or complained; although she had every right to do so. Her strength kept us going.

One day in early May, in fact the day after Sammy shared her ability to "fly", her O2 sats crashed and she was rushed down to PICCU. The oxygen was not enough, and she had to be intubated. Seeing her laying there with a breathing tube down her throat, her chest rising and falling in sequence with the machine at her bedside formed a crack in my heart.

They pumped her full of fluids, her little body swelled more than I could ever imagine. We sat at her bedside, stroking her hand and waited for a miracle. They say that coma patients can hear or at least sense those around them. Although we were uncertain of the accuracy of this belief, we carried on as if it were. We read her books – Peter Pan and Treasure Island and the like. I read motorcycle magazines cover to cover out loud, knowing it was my voice that mattered rather than the content.

The inclusion of the word intensive in PICCU is derived from the nursing content in this unit. Each patient had their own dedicated nurse, for constant monitoring. Leaving together to eat was rare, but having such intense care allowed an occasional meal outside of the hospital. As the days passed our fears grew. We were told that the latest drug they were trying could have serious side effects, including hearing loss and possible developmental issues. Effects that wouldn't happen if she didn't recover, and recovery was all we hoped for. Each additional day of intubation further reduced the odds of recovery; our baby girl was slowly slipping away from us.

On the evening of May 17, our exhaustion began to take over. The nurse assured us that she would call at the first sign of any change and advised us to go back to the House and both get a good night's sleep. We were wearing down. The lack of proper rest would make us susceptible to an illness that would keep us out of the hospital. That was something that simply could not be allowed to happen. The stress and fatigue also wore down our emotional ability to handle our living nightmare. If Sammy was aware of us in those final days, she knew that leaky eyes were much more prominent now that her eyes were closed.

I think it was around 10pm when we settled in at Ronald McDonald House for the last time. The alarm was set for five, and sleep took us quickly. We felt slightly guilty for leaving her, but knew she was in good hands while ours were completely useless now.

The phone woke us just after 4am. Sammy was crashing and we needed to be there. The nurse said she was stable, but to get there soon. Everything is a blur as we grab our clothes and run out the door.

The halls are dim as we speed-walk out of the elevator, heading for PICCU. We aren't even to her room yet when the small light above her door began to flash. Nurses and doctors suddenly appeared from everywhere and rushed into her room. My head exploded with a searing pain worse than a thousand migraines.

Sammy had a massive pulmonary hemorrhage. The blood coming from her breathing tube was the scariest site I had ever seen. I won't describe it any further, more for my own benefit than for yours. They tried to save her but her time with us was over. When the doctors cleared away, they let us hold her for one last time. The crack in my heart that had begun over a week ago widened and I thought I would fall to the floor myself. I clutched her to my chest, her bald head resting below my chin. My daughter had taken flight, leaving her illness behind.

As her blood seeped slowly into my yellow hospital gown, tears flowing down my face onto hers, I had a revelation. In an instant I flashed back to her birth, to that initial terrifying moment when we thought she had left us during her arrival into this world. I remembered the fear and despair that had clutched my heart in a vise for that painful single minute. Now here I stood, almost exactly three years later.

My mind churned constantly as we went upstairs to empty our former room, just as Johnny's father had done. We packed up our few belongings at Ronald McDonald House as well and headed for home, an empty car-seat in the back.

Why? Why had our child been taken from us? Obviously she had done nothing to deserve such a fate, so were we being punished? Had I been right in thinking that I don't deserve to be happy? Had the last few years just been a trick to let my guard down and think that I could have a good life, only to have to my world smashed to pieces again?

It is at times like this when your faith, your belief in an all-knowing and all-powerful being is shaken to the very foundation. If there is any basic truth behind our religion, how could a loving God allow an innocent child to suffer this way? It made no sense. We wanted; we needed to be angry at someone or something. The doctors did their best, we did everything we could, but the end was unacceptable and unavoidable.

The more that I thought about this chain of events, the more it took a different slant. What if we hadn't been robbed of a lifetime with Sammy? What if we were meant to lose her at birth as I had feared that morning three year ago? If that was the case, then the past three years had been a gift. The last nine months had been horrific, but not without good times as well. The memories we made with Sammy in hospital are permanently etched in our souls.

So if we view this as an extension, and we believe as I do that everything happens for a reason; the big question is still why. Was it just to ensure that we appreciate life? Was it to solidify the love we have for our two remaining children and protect them even more from any harm? Or was it to show us that no matter what we do, life will end when it ends, and we should treasure each day while we are here?

It took me awhile to figure it out, but I knew there was a greater purpose here. It was up to me to find that reason. I wasn't going to let Sammy be forgotten.

The next week or two we lived in a thick fog. We were kept busy making arrangements and trying to console Noah and Vicky. I tried to stay focused on one task at a time; keeping moving was essential. I returned Sammy's bicycle; the clerk didn't question the lateness when I mentioned why. I wrote Sammy's eulogy myself; reading it at her funeral was unbelievably difficult. Knowing that she was watching me made it even harder.

Her casket was beautiful, but so tiny. They shouldn't have to make them so small. Despite the comparably small grave, I wanted to crawl down there with her and let them bury me as well. Returning to a life without her seemed impossible. She had been our everything for the past nine months. She was our only concern, our only goal, our only purpose. Now that purpose was gone, so why were we still here?

Obviously we had other children to take care of, but the transition back to a "normal" world or life before was difficult. Although the degree of solace it brings is questionable at best, one of my motto's is "It could have been worse." We knew of couples who had lost their only child to cancer at an equally young age. I couldn't imagine returning to a home completely devoid of children's laughter, to return to being a couple from being a family – that would be worse.

Sammy and Vicky had been genetically identical, raised in identical environments and exposed to the same things. Sammy was taken from us and Vicky left behind. It could have been worse. I honestly do not think I would have had the strength to endure losing two. I am so thankful for having our two children here with us.

That summer we tried to run away from the pain by relocating to a different city. Part of it was a logical escape from the pollution of Chemical Valley where we had been living when Sammy got sick. Sarnia is well known as a hot spot for many cancers including various childhood cancers. I couldn't risk losing another child. Part of it was hoping to avoid the pity-filled looks, and another reason was to escape from everything that reminded us that she was gone. Parks and trips to the local petting zoo brought tears instead of joy. The move was an opportunity and a simple desire to start fresh; a misguided attempt to run from the despair.

The move was successful in one aspect at least; we were kept busy. Preparing the house to sell was actually less effort than any previous move as my mother had been diligently cleaning every inch of it. The main bathroom had been gutted and remodeled to ensure that no mold was hidden behind a once-leaky faucet. A whole-house HEPA filter had been installed to be certain that Sammy wouldn't be exposed to any germs when she returned.

Finding a suitable house in a two day visit was a challenge, but our decision was made that we were moving. My job transfer was fairly easy, but Lori took a few weeks to find the right position. The summer flew by, just as we needed it to. Still, there were those mornings when curling up in the closet and crying all day seemed to be the most pressing thing on the "to-do" list. We tried to stay strong, to stay positive and happy for the kids' sake, but it was not easy.

Noah started his first day of Kindergarten in Cambridge, not knowing a soul. Once again, I worked evenings while Lori worked days and we passed at 3:30 pm each afternoon. The following year I changed jobs, moving to a day-shift. Lori had a job in the accounting department at a daycare in Kitchener, so Victoria started going to daycare there since both of us now worked days. We had established a new routine and tried to settle into it.

I now have to jump back a bit to explain the creation of the fundraiser which appeared to have been my greater purpose.

7 - THE R.O.C.K.

The idea for a memorial ride percolated slowly during that summer as we settled into our new surroundings. My belief that Sammy's death was meant to be the fuel that would drive my purpose was indisputable. How I was to accomplish that goal, through what means I should keep her memory alive was uncertain. A charity ride seemed a logical avenue, so it was down this path I ran, hoping that my choice was true.

In October, I found someone in Burlington willing to design and host our website, the first step in the birth of the R.O.C.K (Ride for Our Cancer Kids). The next step was finding the proper recipient of our funds. After much investigation, we opted for Childhood Cancer Canada with our monies earmarked for the C17 Research Fund. Our funds would end up at the seventeen Children's Hospitals across Canada, including the two that had helped Sammy and become so very near to our hearts.

I printed up a brief bio of Sammy's story and started contacting local companies for prizes and supplies. The response was phenomenal. My employer offered their parking lot for our start and finish. A local printer made a large banner for us and hundreds of colour posters to advertise in the region. Local bike shops provided helmets, jackets, motorcycle luggage and certificates for prizes. We had over six thousand dollars' worth for our top ten fundraisers our first year. A local jeweller who was heavily involved in the biker charity world donated a $2500 diamond ring to be used as our grand prize. Every $50 in donations warranted a rider with a raffle ticket for that ring.

Participation in the event was fairly simple. Riders printed their registration form from our website or obtained it directly from local shops or from us at area events. Then they collected fundraising pledges from friends, family and coworkers. On ride day we collected all the funds, gave them an event t-shirt and set out on our actual ride.

Plotting the route was a major undertaking, but very enjoyable. I spent many afternoons exploring the many scenic rural roads north of Cambridge, in search of a perfect route each year. Primary importance was the safety of our riders. Secondary was including as many beautiful back roads as possible. Many roads had to be dismissed due to a blind intersection or gravel sections.

The first year we had one corner that could not be avoided, but was also a route for gravel trucks heading to some construction. On ride morning, Lori and I drove the route putting up large directional signs that marked the route for our riders. The signs were also donated by a local sign company, and essential for riders without a passenger to constantly watch a printed map. We had some strange looks from the passing vehicles as we swept that intersection at four a.m. Safety was always number one.

That first year we had forty-six riders show up for our inaugural ROCK ride; a decent turnout for a first event but less than we had expected. We had 150 t-shirts on hand and 30 large pizzas ready for a larger crowd. What we didn't expect was the amount of funds raised. We handed over a cheque that day for over thirteen thousand dollars, a phenomenal amount for a first event. The Foundation had a representative on site, the Mayor of Cambridge made a speech; it was a good day.

The next year we changed the venue to a local bar so that we had air conditioning at the Finale. The route was revamped to include the amazing Forks of the Credit Road near Orangeville. Our promotion methods were tweaked and our corporate sponsors grew. That year we had over 80 riders and doubled our proceeds for Childhood Cancer to $26,000. I knew we were on the right path; the R.O.C.K. had become an established event.

After two years in Cambridge, Lori and I started thinking about uprooting it and moving back "home" to Sarnia. The lack of family in close proximity had its down side, and the reasons for leaving seemed less paramount. While the pollution had not changed, my doubts on the cause of Sammy's cancer had increased. While the risks with bph in baby bottles had not yet been realized, there were many other potential cancer causing risks that a simple relocation could not avoid.

There are so many environmental hazards in our industrialized world that avoiding them is nearly impossible. We inject our cattle and chicken with growth hormones and yet wonder why our cells suddenly grow uncontrollably. We spray our vegetables with pesticides that require protective clothing to handle. Our foods contain more chemicals and preservatives than ever before. We spray pesticides in our parks where our infant children crawl around on the ground. Until recently, our playground equipment was saturated with arsenic to preserve the lumber.

It is narrow-minded and naïve to think that we can eliminate all the causes that we know we have created ourselves. The merit of genetically mutated crops that can grow in drier conditions and save millions from famine cannot be overlooked. At the same time, the impact on our own health can be as detrimental as starvation.

The number of chemicals in the list of known carcinogens and those that are potentially cancer causing is huge. If you look deep enough, the number of products which we handle, work with and ingest daily that contain these chemicals is astounding.

While the length of time it takes for a new treatment to become approved and available to the public is shockingly pitiful, new untested products are released daily. The impacts of long-term exposure to various items are largely unknown until the number of deaths warrants an investigation. Sometimes this leads to a ban or restrictions but often it is too engrained in our society to be eliminated.

It is well known that benzene causes cancer, but are we going to eliminate gasoline? The world would grind to a halt if we did; we are nowhere near ready to replace our combustions engine with electric vehicles. Wood dust can cause nasal cancers, but we can't stop the construction industry. Natural elements such as the ultraviolet rays from the sun cause skin cancer, but do we all stay indoors?

Avoiding everything that can cause cancer is as impossible as avoiding anything dangerous. Some people won't fly as they think airplanes are dangerous, but you have a higher chance of being killed in an automobile accident. The paranoid traveller tries to only commute on horseback, but is thrown when his steed is spooked by a snake and breaks his neck in the fall. The steadfast walker is hit by lightning while crossing an open field. There is no avoiding risk.

Mitigating that risk is something that everyone does to different degrees. Some people will only eat organic fruit and vegetables in hopes to avoid the harmful chemicals, despite there being no firm definition or guidelines of being organic. The number of smokers willfully sucking on their cancer sticks has dropped dramatically over the years. Despite the graphic warnings on each pack and the undeniable knowledge that they are flirting with cancer and other diseases, people still light up.

I cannot say with any degree of certainty that Sammy would still be alive if we had moved away from Chemical Valley before her birth. I cannot say if she would be here if I hadn't taken them out to the park behind our house which was chemically weed-controlled. I cannot say that she would be here if the girls had been breast-fed only, thus avoiding the plastic bottles laced with bph at the time. I cannot say that she would be here if we hadn't put flea powder on our dog that she loved to pet. I simply do not know, and never will.

Living in a bubble is not an option and is not living. Our daily dangers have changed over the millennia. We don't live in fear of wild animals venturing into our caves. We can not only survive, but even flourish despite being inept at hunting or gathering berries. We have developed into a race that creates our own dangers as we strive to make our lives better.

That summer I decided that I could make a better life for my family by moving back to Sarnia, despite the risk of the petrochemical pollution that would surround us. It was not an easy decision, but just as I did not regret moving away, I do not regret coming back. Both moves were critical in my path and both had to take place in their own time.

Lori was able to get back in with her previous employer up the road and I took an evening supervisor position at another local broker. A few months later I was offered a job at a large broker as Branch Manager, where I stayed for the next six years.

Some of our previous sponsors stayed on board despite the 200 km move. Many new sponsors came on board right away, so we weren't really back to square one. A few riders continued making the trek down for future years and we actively promoted the ride locally. Although we were in a smaller population centre, there were fewer events to compete with.

In our first year in Sarnia, the success of the event was comparable with the last year in Cambridge. For the next four years, we hovered near $30,000 raised with around a hundred riders participating. In 2011 we jumped to 38,000 with still just under a hundred participants. The website was switched over to a third party provider connected with the Foundation. It was a template format which I could modify myself while maintaining our rockride.com domain. Riders could now pre-register online and raise funds months before the event with electronic tax receipts issued instantly. Our event was maturing.

In 2012, we reached our "Quarter Million Raised to Date" milestone; an impressive achievement in just nine years. Each year we made some changes to keep it fresh, but our planning process was established and we were well known as a well-organized, fun and worthwhile charity ride.

Along the way, we met some great people that had also been touched by childhood cancer. Touched is far from an accurate term to describe the impact, but it will suffice for now. One of our top fundraisers every year was the father of a survivor named Julia. He worked for Canada Customs at the border where I worked, although we didn't really know each other until her diagnosis at eleven months of age. Her chances of recovery were far worse than Sammy's original prognosis, but she made it. Her family has become part of the event, hosting a pre-ride bbq at the bridge in Sarnia each year, even after they moved to a different city.

Another young survivor that I feel the need to mention is young Zoe. It was at our 2011 event when I became aware of her battle, although I didn't actually meet her that day.

On ride day, busy doesn't begin to describe me. There are a hundred things going on and I need to keep my thumb on all of them. The event is very well planned out but I always feel pulled in multiple directions at any one moment. I enjoy it immensely. I thrive on being busy and each event is a highlight that is eagerly anticipated.

That morning, a soft-spoken gentleman named Jeff introduced himself at registration. Our conversation was brief, but he wanted to thank me personally for all we were doing for the cause and handed me a sealed envelope to look at later, when I had a minute. I thanked him and stuffed the card into the inner pocket of my leather vest.

The event went off without a hitch, and eight hours later I noticed the envelope still in my vest pocket. I had ridden home alone; Lori and the kids were following in the van, loaded with materials from the Finale. They must have stopped to grab something to eat as I was home for a solid fifteen minutes before them.

I was glad that I hadn't pulled the envelope out on stage to read while waiting for the band to wrap up. The ride is always a very emotional day and my speech tops off the day. It is always well received, but I am always completely drained at the end. The card inside that envelope pushed me over the edge and I sat down and bawled uncontrollably for some time.

The card had a hand-drawn picture on the front of a young bald girl standing in a field of flowers with "Thank You!" along the bottom and the sub-text "Love Zoe -8 yrs. old 2010". It appeared to be a card made in the hospital and copies created by one of the organizations that work with the children doing crafts and the like.

On the left inner page, her parents had written, "Thank you so much for all your hard work organizing the rockride! My daughter Zoe was diagnosed with ovarian cancer July 15 of last year. Six rounds of chemo and lots of love and support… she is doing great! I want you to know that what you do saves lives like my Zoe's. We are truly grateful and cannot thank you enough!"

On the opposing page, the message from Zoe was written in four different coloured gel-pen inks. "Thank you 4 raising lots of money 4 kid's cancer. From Zoe. The "o" in Zoe was replaced with a heart.

This simple and heart-felt card had a huge impact on me that day. It is one of the mementos that I will keep forever. The following year her father signed up under "Team Zoe". This very special motorcycle club of one ended up winning our Club Cup for the next two years. While the Club Cup trophy was created in Cambridge when we had a larger number of actual clubs in the area to compete for it, the number of riders from the local groups had been very limited. The criteria to win was simply the most money raised by attending members of that group or club, so a single man had the potential to win over a half a dozen riders who raised less pledges.

The highlight of all our events to date was our tenth anniversary ride in 2013. It was a near perfect day, despite a route change the week before due to an unexpected construction detour.

The adjustment threatened to break up our group as we were now going through a series of traffic lights which we would normally avoid. Our rural routes were carefully planned to avoid impacting traffic without the need for police escorts or costly road closures. Somehow, all eighty-five bikes stayed together for most of the return run from our midpoint bbq hosted by a local Optimist group. As we crested the overpass, I looked back and all I could see were bikes. It is an impressive site and one I look forward to each year.

The actual highlight was an unexpected performance at the Finale by my daughter, Victoria. I had written a song two years earlier about losing Samantha and the birth of the R.O.C.K. but she had been unable to sing it at the 2011 ride. Earlier in the year, she had sung it at a talent show at her school, but felt that she would get too emotional at this year's ride and be unable to get through singing it.

Victoria was riding with me as a passenger that day, as she often did. Partway through the route, she told me that she was thinking about singing the song I had written at our awards ceremony rather than the Our Lady Peace song that was planned. I told her that would be great if she could and not a big deal if she found herself unable to do so at the last minute. I didn't want to pressure her and knew that she was nervous.

I still was unsure which song she would perform when I introduced her at the beginning of our Finale presentation. I was filled with pride when she started with, "I'm going to do a song that my Dad wrote. It's called Three Years. I hope you like it."

> *Twin girls were born on a warm May morn, filling my world with joy.*
> *Daily troubles and silent fears left at the door, as I watched you dance with glee around the floor.*
> *I rode home each day to hear this beloved stereo.*
>
> *Three years I held your hand,*

WE MUST CARRY ON

Three years you were my world,
Two years of heaven and one of hell.
I see your image every day, and miss you every hour, Now,
just a ghostly apparition in my mirror.

Hearts shattered as the word echoed down the hall, Bottles
'n soothers now chemo and scans.
You whispered, "Don't cry Daddy, no leaky eye,"
Oh, my baby, everyday - I still try.

Three years I held your hand,
Three years you were my world,
Two years of heaven and one of hell.
I see your image every day, and miss you every hour, Now,
just a ghostly apparition in my mirror.

On a cold May night, you gained your wings.
Tears soaked my bloodstained gown as I held you tight.
Nine months you fought, never losing your spirit, I pray I
have your strength, for I miss you so.

Three years I held your hand,
Three years you were my world,
Two years of heaven and one of hell.
I see your image every day, and miss you every hour, Now,
just a ghostly apparition in my mirror.

Rumbling down the blacktop, a hundred bikes in my wake,
Images of you flash past like streetlights in my mind.
You fly above me, watching me as I watched you.
We ride for you, we ride with you... In my mirror.

The video of her performance is likely still out there, posted on YouTube.

BOB THOMAS

8 - INTERLUDE – YOUR PATH

For a while I thought the R.O.C.K. was my fated path. The logic was undeniable. Samantha was given a life extension as a means to an end. That end, we hope, will be a break-through in cancer research that is made possible, at least in part, by the funds we raise each year. Or maybe it's more convoluted, but just as sequential. Maybe a young person reads about Samantha and decides to study oncology, eventually being that key person with that much needed discovery. Our event is keeping her memory alive and her story maintained in the media.

How it will happen, I do not know. Some things you must take on faith. Even in hindsight, the sequence of events is not always apparent, but the chain of events is there none the less. My belief in a sequential pattern to life is not to say that I think that our fates are predetermined. In fact, it is our free will that makes our lives worth living. The possible futures are endless and every decision we make is another fork in the road that leads us down a complex interwoven matrix of limitless possibilities.

Sometimes you may look back and think that you made a wrong decision that put you back to square one on what you believe to be your life path. Let's consider Jill for a moment. She decides to attend University upon graduation from high school, majoring in English Literature as she has always had a passion for books and considers herself an "Academic". Ten years later, she finds herself dissatisfied at her job as a fact-checker at a local newspaper. Her fiancé has a child from a previous marriage, who happens to have autism. Jill has formed a close bond with the child and yearns to know more about treatment for the illness.

As "luck" would have it, her fiancé gets a promotion at work that gives them the financial freedom for Jill to go back to school to study psychology. Ten years later Jill develops a new therapy that has a significant impact on the communication skills in nearly half of the mid-level autistic children that completed her program.

One could say that her literary degree and subsequent work at the newspaper was a waste of time. Those years were a circular path with no relevant outcome. It was not until she started school a second time, on her true path, that she really made a difference.

From a different standpoint however, she was not at the right point in her life to proceed down that "true" path. She had not had the opportunity to meet her fiancé or his son. She had not realized the importance of a work that she had not even considered. Her arguably unnecessary education still gave her the tools to analyse theories and interpret hidden meanings. Young people often fail to realize that much of education, especially in the elementary levels, is to teach you how to learn rather than to teach you specific things.

There is no singular path for each of us to follow, but rather a plethora of possible futures. Sometimes we find ourselves drawn to a particular path despite conscious attempts to head down a different one. Is that a result of our own subconscious, a genetic predisposition that has seeped in from the foundation built by our parents, or an omnipotent power? That question we can leave to the philosophy students for now.

All that you need to know is that everyone has futures available to them. Find your path, change your path if needed, but keep moving forward. The world is ever changing, and every change has some impact on your surroundings. Take advantage of the positive changes and discard the negatives.

Life is not always easy, and the path to a happy and meaningful life will not always seem happy or meaningful. Your path may be twisted and bumpy and you may feel completely lost at times. Even once you find your chosen path, or you may think you have, it may be suddenly blocked by a huge boulder that seems too huge to navigate around.

Just as various jobs can be stepping stones in your career, these boulders that appear along your path can actually become stepping stones to propel you along your life path. The trick is not allowing them to stop your ever-forward momentum. Climbing over that obstacle builds your muscles and strengthens your resolve. Standing on top of that boulder can provide an entirely new perspective and allow you to see the path before you. We have all heard the saying, "You can't see the forest for the trees". The obstacle can provide the opportunity to rise above the tree line and see the forest for a moment.

Losing Samantha was a huge boulder that fell from the sky and nearly crushed me. Finding the strength to climb that rock and jump forward to a new meaningful future was unbelievably hard. I wanted to curl up in its shadow, hidden from the world and wait to wither away. The hardships faced in my youth which I thought had made me weak and broken had actually made me stronger. It was touch and go for a while but I was able to see past the anger and despair and continue moving forward.

During Sammy's illness, nothing else mattered. The threat of losing our child really put all the little things in perspective. I thought about all the daily stresses and problems that can make you lose sleep and worry. None of them seemed even remotely relevant when a real problem like this appeared.

Perspective – the one thing that we have trouble keeping a grip on. We get upset because our auto repair bill is high. We get angry because a co-worker gets a bonus despite being a complete slacker. We worry about what others think about our new hairstyle. None of it matters.

Youth seem to have the biggest problem getting the proper perspective and adults have the biggest problem understanding their lack of it. Imagine fifteen year old Jane for a moment. Her first boyfriend Jack has just dumped her. In her eyes, the world has ended. She thinks that she will never love or be loved again. In reality, their six week relationship was merely infatuation, puppy love, nothing more. She starts to question her appearance. Jack's new "girlfriend" is skinnier and has longer hair. Jane starts to skip meals when her parents don't notice. She spends hours staring in the mirror, obsessing over her acne and still barely noticeable breasts.

Her grades start to drop alongside her self-confidence. She gets in a fight after school with a friend of Jack's new girlfriend. She is completely oblivious to the affectionate glances from Peter whose locker is just three down from her own. Her parents' period of soft consoling and understanding has long since ended. Her poor attitude and obsessive behaviours only anger them now. Their comments push her farther away. "He was just a boy. You're only fifteen and don't even know what love is. Get over it already."

She has lost all perspective, and her parents have forgotten how fragile a young girl's heart can be. Relationships, no matter how brief they may be can have a significant impact on a developing psyche. Losing someone close to us, even if it is just the end of that bond rather than an actual life, can be very difficult. Even a short-term relationship can be extremely hard to cope with for many people. Time does indeed heal most wounds, but we tend to be an impatient species, wanting immediate fulfillment.

Those of us with low self-esteem tend to expect that we will never find another person as good as the one we just lost. Usually we feel this way not because we truly believe that person was perfect but because we feel unworthy of anyone perceived to be of such a high calibre. This lack of hope can lead to depression at an already vulnerable period of time. The key again is hope, perspective and the realization that not only are there plenty of fish in the sea, but we are worthy of being loved by someone.

Some people think that there is a single soul-mate out there for them. Such a belief can set you up for a devastating sense of loss if you lose that person once they have been found. In reality, there are hundreds of potential relationships out there. Everything is complicated however, as we are all at different stages in our own personal development or evolution. Often relationships do not work out simply because the two people involved are moving in different directions as that particular point.

In today's world, we tend to move through different partners as we learn about ourselves and fashion our own likes and dislikes. Being exposed to varying personalities can be paramount in our own development. In other cases, a couple may bond at a relatively young age and develop together. This is not to say that they are robbing themselves of the opportunity to experience other people and how other relationships could work or not work. Every person is different and every interaction is different. My point here would be not to judge, but always support those around you.

I was lucky in finding my wife when I did. I was starting a new chapter in my life and we developed together over the years. Many marriages don't survive the loss of a child, but we did. Many would not have survived the difficulties that come with sexual abuse or the recovery of repressed memories. It was a bumpy ride, but we are still together. I consider that proof that love can conquer all, even if that love often feels undeserved.

To be honest, I sincerely doubt if I would have been able to continue this far along my path without my wife. The undertow in my ocean of despair likely would have sucked me back under if she hadn't been up on my board waiting for me. If another room in my house had remained empty, I likely would have went back down the hall to a former home and lived there in despair. Instead we kept our paths intertwined and have come further along our paths together than we could have managed alone; of that I am certain.

Lately I began to wonder if raising awareness and funds for childhood cancer may not have been my final destination after all.

Although its importance is never in question, maybe I need to keep moving forward. Building the event has forced me outside of my comfort zone, transforming into a better person. I proved to myself that I am confidant and capable enough to transform loss into gain. Maybe I am supposed to also turn my previous life-altering hardship into something positive as well. So now I sit here, sharing my story in hopes that you can learn from it. Maybe someone will read this book and change their way of thinking. Someone may propel themselves up the surface and alter their perspective of life. Someone may dip their arm into the water below and pull another troubled soul to the surface.

It's doubtful that I would ever know such an effect took place; that I helped save a life just by documenting and sharing my life thoughts. I will proceed though, on the chance that I could be helping others. I will keep moving forward. I will have faith that my path is valid and justified.

9 - TRUTHS REVEALED

The old adage "when it rains, it pours" was never a more understated comment than it was for me in 2002. The stress from Samantha's illness was unrelenting, but we had no inclination that she would not recover. Lori was staying in the London hospital with her when the real memories began to surface. I couldn't share my recollections at the time; my mental trauma was insignificant at the time and adding to my wife's burden would be as cruel as it would be non-productive.

I had firmly believed that I had been spared any abuse from my father. There was not a single ounce of doubt about it. The lack of abuse had troubled me for years though. Why was I left unscathed from the nightmare? Not that having a pedophile for a father can really leave one undamaged, but you get my meaning.

That fall, my exhaustion led to a breach in my memory vault that was hidden in the deepest darkest corner of my mind. I had built that safe so well and hidden it so deeply that I did not even remember that it existed. The cracks deepened and the memories that I dared not accept as truth began to surface.

I had long ago given up the idea of a remote chance that Dad had died an innocent man. That would have been a different but equally terrible truth to live with. Regardless of that certainty, the actual memories of abuse were very difficult to process.

While this chapter should warrant more in depth discussion, I am not ready or able to delve too deeply at this point. I was able to come to terms with much of it over time and with some professional help. I will share a few memories and realizations however, for this boulder is part of who I am. The fact that it is relevant for some who may be reading this, distresses me greatly.

This particular memory came to me gradually, through a series of dreams which eventually ended further along the timeline. While it was not part of my abuse, it was proof of Dad's twisted mind and I had subconsciously thrown this memory into my secret vault.

It was early spring with snow still covering much of the road into the track. My bike was covered in mud by the time I made it down to our office-trailer. Nobody had been down to the track for weeks. One could access it by snowmobile through the winter but now the snow was too sporadic for sleds yet too much for regular vehicles.

It was colder than I expected, so I was stopping at the trailer to search for an additional layer of clothing before resuming my ride. I searched all the drawers and cupboards but to no avail. The only other spot that we might have something stashed was under the beds at the back. There were sliding door-covers on either side of the wheel for extra storage. It was impressive how much usable space they managed to design into these small trailers.

I awoke at this point the first couple times I had this dream. I remembered it when I awoke and quickly realized that this was not a random dream but a real memory. This had happened to me in real life, without a doubt. I didn't fully realize that it was a forgotten memory: I just had never thought about it before. If someone had asked, "Do you remember that spring when you rode into the track through the mud and were looking for extra gloves?" I thought I would have said yes, but now I wonder if I would have remembered if asked, or was it secured in the vault until now?

The next time I dreamt further on in time. Behind the panel was a bundle of magazines, pornographic magazines. The top couple were Playboy and Hustler, standard magazines for the eighties. Further down were magazines with strange names, although I can't recall them now. The cover of the first obscene magazine had a picture of a young boy, completely nude except for a Peter Pan style hat. His hand was covering his genitals. He didn't look to be more than ten or eleven years old. Then I awoke.

The next time I recalled this memory, it included the sound of dad's tractor coming down the hill to the track. I remember feeling ashamed for having looked at the magazines. I don't recall feeling any shock or surprise at seeing the non-traditional material though.

The last time I had that dream; it only lasted a few moments more. Dad entered the trailer just as I was jamming the bundle of magazines back into the hiding place beneath the bunk. He asked if I had been looking at our magazines. The pronoun in that sentence and the green Robin Hood style cap on the cover were the two most prominent things that I remember. Mercifully I awoke at that point, and whatever happened or did not happen after that moment remains securely in the vault.

Another prominent dream that caused many restless nights was part memory and part fantasy. I know the latter half was fantasy, an alternate path not taken, for it was not I who took Dad's life. This recurring dream was not something that leaked from my vault, but began to manifest as I came to realize my early first-hand knowledge of my father's reprehensible actions.

Dad and I were walking alone through the woods. The ground was covered in leaves, still wet from an early morning shower. It was definitely autumn but whether or not it was really deer season or not was hard to say. We owned a large enough plot of land that the odds of getting caught hunting out of season were miniscule. When times were tough, filling our freezer with fresh venison was par for the course, regardless of the time of year.

I was carrying Dad's Winchester rifle, following him carefully through the forest. I was only ten or eleven at the time and had only shot the 30.30 a couple times. The kids mainly stuck to the 22 calibre single shot for target practice.

In reality, we came to an old fence that was partially fallen down. Dad circled back when I hollered and took the rifle from me so I could carefully step over. In my dream, that part ended differently. Every night for quite some time that dream ended differently.

In my dream, I knew that he was a monster in disguise. In my dream, I quickly deduced that the authorities would determine the shooting to be an accident. A young boy, who should have never been carrying a loaded fire-arm, snagged his foot on an unseen piece of fence and the weapon went off. Tragically, the boy's father was killed in the incident. There would be no thorough investigation that might uncover a motive.

Dad had stopped a few metres ahead to let me catch up, scanning the woods ahead for movement. I slowly took off the safety and took aim at his spine. I quietly mouthed the words, "No more" and squeezed the trigger. Some nights the gunshot woke me, while others I saw him crumple to the ground.

This dream led to quite a bit of "what if" thinking for a while. It also tied in heavily with the recurring "circle of accusers" dream that came years later. Indeed, if I had had the strength of will at the time I could have saved many from his abuse. I will never know exactly how many victims he had, but I fear that number could be high. He certainly had many opportunities over the years, and the math just seems to add up too easily in many of those cases.

If I had really pulled that trigger, my life would have completely different – I think. The track never would have been completed and then foreclosed on. I would never have succumbed to depression and recovered from my downward spiral by moving south to start over. Or would the three of us have returned to Sarnia where Mom had family to help out? Would the same course of events still have eventually played out if I had killed the monster in my youth? I'll never know.

I frequently joke that my time machine is broken. If I had the ability to go back and relive that moment, what would I do? Knowing what I know now, would I risk changing my life completely? Would I potentially sacrifice my future in order to save an unknown number of victims? Although I sincerely doubt I would have been institutionalized for the killing, it would definitely have had an impact. Most people would not have realized that he deserved to die. The secret likely never would have seen the light of day. I would have been pitied for a different reason; I would be that poor little kid who accidentally shot his own father.

Logically I do not blame myself for not pulling the trigger. I did not consciously know of the abuse at that point. My memories were already locked away and the existence of a key long since forgotten. Even if I had known, I was just a kid; a timid child with no violent tendencies. I know that nobody holds me responsible for my father's crimes.

My subconscious however, does not always think logically and reasonably. This is clearly indicated in the recurring dream that led me to the Sexual Assault Survivor Centre and ultimately to the creation of this book. The dream haunted me nightly, trying to push me down into the murky depths of depression once again.

Everyone whom Dad had ever abused stood in a circle around me. Actually they weren't really standing, as we were all floating in a black abyss. The lack of natural light didn't conceal them, for they had an eerie fluorescence that grew brighter as each moved closer to me. The theme of their messages was as singular as it was demanding. Their accusations illogical to a rational mind, but obviously embedded in my subconscious, for that was their true point of origin.

"Why did you let him do that to me?"

"Why didn't you stop him?"

"Why couldn't you please him, so he'd stop coming to me?"

"Why didn't you tell someone?"
"I thought you were my friend."
"You could have prevented this, you had the chance."
"He may have been a monster, but you're a coward."
"It's your fault."

At some point in their barrage, I would break down in tears or scream in defiance, only to awake and realize that I was safe in my bed.

We can strive to be logical and reasonable, but our emotions and our screwed up psychological baggage can lead to some very irrational thoughts and reactions. Re-training that instinctual side to be rational, or finding the patience to delay a reaction until you can think it through, is no small task. In a world of instantaneous gratification and immediate responses, that knee-jerk reaction is often the one that is shown. If your inner demons have damaged your core to the point where it is rarely rational, you must consciously work to control your reactions. Slow yourself down and allow adequate time to process things through the level-headed and sensible part of yourself.

Some people say they strive to live with "no regrets". This is not a realistic goal in my opinion. Regret is a feeling of disappointment over something that has happened. This is completely normal and unavoidable. The key is not obsessing over it and learning from the experience. A simple regret like, "I wish I hadn't yelled at my son last night," is easily corrected with an apology and a conscious effort to remain calm the next time.

In a broad scope, most people tend to regret more things that they didn't do rather than those they did. Haven't we all looked back at the previous year or decade and wished we had found more time to travel, to visit with family? I think the idea of a bucket list is a great concept. The key there once again is to put in not only meaningful items but also realistic ones. Travelling around the world is likely not an attainable goal for many people. Financial limitations and obligations make some things almost impossible without major ramifications. One can't abandon their family, quit their job and cash in all their pension savings just so they can cross that item off their list. Set reasonable goals and try to cross off at least one item each year. Once you have the momentum started, reaching your goals will become easier.

Regret, just like anything else, can be a source of negative or positive energy. Learn from your mistakes, whether big or small. Living in the past means not moving forward and momentum is absolutely essential when it comes to following your path, whatever path you choose it to be.

Over the years I reached out to a variety of "professionals" to help with my issues. The earliest being non-voluntary after the truth came out and Dad was charged. The resulting anti-depressants helped me sleep, but I don't recall any other real benefit. The world around me was falling apart, but I didn't really start falling apart until much later, so maybe they did help.

Before I came to my own personal realizations regarding my past, I pro-actively sought help with another condition which I eventually realized is likely related to my abuse as well. To date, I still have not overcome this particular issue. I had high hopes that the realization of the underlying psychological reason would miraculously eliminate the physical manifestations from which I still suffer.

I suffer from S.E.D. – Selective Eating Disorder. There are very few foods that I can eat without triggering my hyperactive gag reflex. Growing up I was described as a picky eater whose parents must not have been strict enough to force the issue. This is like saying that someone with the Coprolalia aspect of Tourette syndrome sometimes uses profanity. My diet consists of what most people would consider childhood foods – French fries, hot dogs, some cookies, crackers and dry cereal.

There seems to be no rhyme or reason as to which foods will trigger my gagging; no specific texture or taste guidelines. How things are prepared is just as vital, not that there is much preparation involved with the foods that I am able to consume. My fries can be deep-fried or baked in the oven, but fresh-cut style with skin left renders them unacceptable. Hot dogs are boiled, without a bun to go along them. Potato chips must be plain, no extra flavouring to spoil the taste. Fruits are limited to apples and bananas, with vegetables being banned from my diet outside of the base potato content in my staple food of course. There are a few other snack foods but my primary sustenance can be counted on a single hand.

I have been this way as long as I can remember, although my mother told me that I used to eat some other foods until I was five or so, then the gagging started. My dietary issues further complicated my social awkwardness. Birthday parties usually included pizza and cake, neither of which I could digest. One father became furious at my rude behaviour in not having any cake at his son's party. He insisted that I grow up and try some. His persistence resulted in vomit on his shoes.

The social impact of my undiagnosed, and at that time un-named, problem continues on to this day. Everything from business luncheons to weddings and casual dinner invitations become awkward and avoided when possible. As years went by, I became more willing to explain that I had what was essentially an eating disorder. If I could avoid the meal without significant repercussions though, feigning an upset stomach or showing up late was usually easier.

Physically my diet has had minimal impact on my health however. My body has adapted accordingly, drawing every bit of nutrition from what I do eat. Although my metabolism has slowed slightly since turning forty, I am traditionally slightly under-weight. This surprises most people when they hear of my French fry diet. My excellent cholesterol numbers and low end blood pressure is a source of envy for the health conscious around me.

Regardless of my current health conditions, I wish I could overcome this disorder. I would give anything to walk into a restaurant and have a steak, or even a hamburger off the barbecue.

Medical doctors could find no physiological reason for my hyperactive gag reflex. One acupressure therapist that I tried after moving to Sarnia had an interesting hypothesis on the root cause of my disorder. I took this theory to heart and used it as my explanation for many people whom I felt deserved a reason for my social rudeness.

Immediately upon hearing of my uncontrollable gag reflex he asked if I had ever had salmonella poisoning. I thought this to be an odd question, but was truly surprised as his inquiry was justified. I had indeed had a life-threatening experience when I was four years old. We had a pet turtle at the time that we had rescued from the lake. Although I see no inherent logic to the action now, I would frequently pet the turtle. While it seemed an inherently inconsequential activity, the results were nearly catastrophic when added to a child's propensity to put unwashed fingers in their mouths. I spent three days in the hospital and apparently flat-lined at one point, or so I am told.

The therapist explained to me that salmonella can do significant damage to the soft palate that triggers the gag reflex. While he could not explain why certain foods were immune from this involuntary response, this was the first scientific theory I had heard to date. He believed that with his acupressure treatments he could trigger some regeneration of the palate and hopefully overcome my affliction.

The treatments failed but acquiring a medical reason for my "pickiness" was worth the cost of the sessions. At various times I tried other alternatives, including hypnosis and acupuncture, with no success. My diet has not changed in over three decades, not a single new food added to my tolerated menu.

During this quest however, I made significant progress in another area. I had stumbled across a new age practitioner who used a variety of methods including acupuncture and regression therapy. I attended a seminar in Kitchener that simply blew my mind. His presentation included muscle-testing with the subjects being exposed to different elements and foods that he claimed they were allergic to.

Despite my initial cynicism, the display proved interesting to say the least.

I set up an appointment to further investigate his belief that he may be able to help me. At this point I had already come to the realization that my gagging could be completely psychological; a result of my traumatic abuse as a child. Both theories seemed plausible, but the mere acknowledgement had not spontaneously eliminated the physical reaction.

Over the course of a couple months we had five or six sessions. We discussed my past in deeper detail than I had ever shared with anyone, including myself. We tried acupuncture twice, which I highly recommend. The relaxed state of being far surpassed anything that I had experienced, even during my brief foray into the world of illicit drugs. The regression therapy sessions left me drained, but peaceful by the end. The random anger that I had fought to hide subsided. Once again, my eating disorder was unchanged, but the treatments worthwhile.

I basically gave up trying to find a "cure" for my problem after that. I focused on our fundraiser and living a normal life for the next few years. I didn't seek any help again until that recurring dream, with the circle of victims blaming me for their abuse. I knew it was irrational but they wouldn't stop their nightly tirade through my subconscious. I teetered on the brink of depression but quickly reached out. Male victims were fairly uncommon at the Sexual Assault Survivors Centre, but I was welcomed just the same.

Biweekly meetings helped me to work through some issues and made me realize how well I actually was handling everything. The latest recurring dream became less frequent and stopped altogether shortly thereafter.

One unexpected benefit of attending the Centre was making contact with one of the ladies who also worked at a local junior high school. The school was having a week of activities focused on teen suicide, drug abuse and mental health issues. Upon learning of my past and my success in overcoming my numerous problems, she approached me about being a guest speaker.

I was nervous to say the least, but felt this could be a vital step in turning the negatives in my past into a positive in the present. I was hesitant in part because I had only discussed my abuse with a very select few. Telling a room full of strangers that I was sexually abused was terrifying. Although we did not know anyone who had children attending the school, the chance that it would leak back to people we did know was nerve-wracking.

After much thought, and after a discussion with my own children, I decided to proceed. Although my speech would focus on overcoming depression and making the conscious decision not to commit suicide, it touched on my abuse, brief substance abuse and Dad's own suicide. Previously my children had been told that my father had died in a car accident. There was a slight element of truth in that statement; he had died in a car. They took the news fairly well, reacting with empathy for the abuse I endured and pride that I was going to use it to help others.

I had scheduled a couple hours off work for an appointment on the day of the speech, arriving early to the school. The gymnasium was set up with chairs for close to four hundred students and staff. I reviewed my speech notes nervously as everyone filed in.

A young woman and her boyfriend spoke before me, which was a relief. They were both recovering drug addicts at the young age of seventeen. I don't believe either of them had spoken in a forum of this size before, but did a great job. Even at a junior high, many of the children seemed to relate to their story of peer pressure, boredom and gateway drugs. I sincerely hope that those boys and girls remember that story when they are offered their first joint or pill.

The room was equally quiet for my speech. I told them briefly of my youth and that I was sexually abused. I shared my suicide attempts after Dad killed himself and my decision to move here to start over. I told them of Sammy's illness and how difficult it was to handle the death of a child. Once the sorrow had sunken in, I shared my recovery and rebirth. I told them of the success of the fundraiser in Sammy's memory and my own personal success that far exceeded anything I would have hoped for in my youth. I stressed the importance of perspective and perseverance; hammering home that everyone is capable of good works.

Following the question and answer period the students were given comment cards which we were allowed to read afterwards. I had not expected any feedback so I was pleasantly surprised. I expected my only reward would be belief that I had touched at least one child that day. One young abused soul that might come forward to stop it; one mind lost in despair that might think twice before pulling the trigger or slashing their wrists. If I had provided some grain of hope to a single person that day, then it was worthwhile.

Skimming through the pencilled comments was an uplifting experience. They seemed very appreciative of our honesty and courage in sharing our obviously uncomfortable histories.

The experience started me thinking about repeating the presentation at other schools, so I shared my willingness with my contact at the Centre. Nothing else came directly from that avenue, but I later hooked up with another charitable group that had just opened a "Suicide Prevention Resource Centre". I met some great people there and had a lot of fun helping with their Haunted House Fundraisers and the like. We never made it as far as arranging presentations at area schools but one never knows what the future may bring.

My hopes are that sharing my story via the written word will be the appropriate conduit to reach those in need. When you are finished this, please feel free to pass it along. One never knows if your copy will reach the hands that really need it.

As we approach the end of our journey through my life to date, it is fitting that we enter a world of post-life influence. Many of you will discard my beliefs or at least some of them. I do not blame you for your cynicism as I was also a non-believer until recently. I waged an inner battle on whether or not to include this portion of my story.

My trepidation was not because I feared criticism or ridicule for this commentary. Just as I was hesitant to begin the book for fear of hurting my family who tried hard to bury the abuse in the past; I hesitated on this portion for fear of the impact on my daughter, Victoria.

I never completely discounted others' belief in anything that could not be scientifically proven. Whether or not I believed had no relevance on the legitimacy of another's belief. My mother's unequivocal faith in God gave her the strength to endure both her illness which eventually took her life, and the mental anguish that came with the horrors of our past. I am not saying that her beliefs were misguided, far from it. What I am saying is that her faith gave her strength when she needed it. That kind of faith, whether it is justified or not, has merit and is of extreme benefit.

There are many things in this world that cannot be explained scientifically, at least not at the present time. We demand to see proof or at least be provided with a logical argument before we believe something is true. The power of man as a species is in our intellect, so a refusal to accept any random statement as gospel truth without some justification is not necessarily a bad thing. At the same time, completely discounting a theory simply because it cannot currently be proven can be narrow-minded.

I'm not going to delve into the eventual proving or disproving of scientific theories, but keep in mind all the things that were once accepted as fact but later completely disproven. No, the world is not flat. Keep in mind other beliefs that have been instilled by society but were later questioned and now seem preposterous. Testing a woman to determine if she is a witch requires drowning – if she lives then she must be a witch.

While we demand proof for some things, others are accepted without reproach. These are usually spiritual in nature, the existence of which should not be questioned or risk being deemed an atheist. The beliefs passed down over the generations have been modified slightly as our society evolves, as they should. Believers are normally given a certain degree of not only tolerance but complete acceptance. The premise of "I don't share your beliefs but you are free to believe as you like, and I won't mock you for it" is a common practice.

While spirituality is considered acceptable, the belief in spirits is still considered fanciful and not widely accepted. People like to believe that their loved ones have gone to a better place. We like to believe that they live on in our hearts and even claim to sometimes feel their presence. However, if someone tells you that they can speak to the deceased, would you believe?

Many people now consider themselves to be spiritual despite not agreeing with much of the doctrines of organized religion. Many people do not attend church or read the bible but they believe in life after death. Every individual is entitled to their beliefs and the power that belief brings can be phenomenal. I can't really say with any conviction what I really believed when it came to life after death. That recently changed though.

I am not sharing this aspect of my life with you in an effort to make you believe. Hearing another's story is rarely sufficient to make a leap of faith and believe that the story is completely factual. Previously I would have written off such a declaration as imaginative and entertaining but not necessarily real. I wasn't so cynical as to think that those who professed stories such as this were actually lying. One can absolutely believe something is real when it is not, of that I am absolutely certain. The mind can play tricks and some illusions are not consciously created, only interpreted incorrectly.

Regardless, my beliefs in certain aspects of the supernatural have certainly changed over the past year. I still question them at times, and do not disagree that some things are not really hard evidence as much as they are interpretations. Overall though, I cannot offer any other reasonable explanation. Just because an explanation may not seem reasonable to some, does not mean that it is not true.

I should also caution that a certain degree of skepticism is not a bad thing. Just as the liars and "players" at a singles bar may deceive and mislead to get what they want, so do the charlatans and fakers in the world of psychics and mediums. I do not like the term "fortune-teller" as it implies a glimpse into the future and your future has not been set. There are many possible paths ahead of you; which path you follow is your decision, for you always have free will. Some mediums may share information using tarot cards, a crystal ball or mere touch. These are all just tools to communicate with another plain of reality.

I am by no means an expert on this subject, so I can only comment on my experiences and beliefs, as limited as they may be. I was told that I will begin a spiritual enlightenment that will alter my perceptions. By the time you read this, maybe I will have a greater understanding of what lies beyond.

While the information received from a local medium was mainly correct, this is not the reason for inclusion in this book. Her knowledge of my personal and private history was unsettling but also set the stage for my belief in spiritual guides. More importantly, that shift opened the door for communication with my daughter Victoria.

Vicky had been "seeing" spirits for some time but had been scared to tell us. The medium had told us that Victoria was extremely gifted and had great potential. She was destined for great things but would need our support. The collaborating information from both sources further strengthened my belief in the psychic connection.

Samantha is indeed with us, and communicates with us through Victoria. My devout mother was hesitant to come through at first, but eventually has admitted that her disbelief in such things was wrong. She is usually the first to reach out when the lines of communication are opened.

This year at the ROCK, we were lined up to leave our midpoint barbeque. There were over eighty motorcycles set up on the road to follow me back to the finale. A few minutes before I gave the signal to mount up, Victoria received a warning from my mother's spirit. We had planned to leave promptly at one o'clock. Mom told her that we had to delay by ten minutes; we absolutely could not leave on time. Vicky told me later that she saw a vision of an accident. There were multiple bikes lying on the highway, and we were among the seriously injured.

We all have those moments of vague premonitions, even if they are on a subconscious level. It's usually just a feeling, a last minute decision to take a different route home or to not take a trip. We write them off as being random acts, but on a subconscious level we know there is danger. This was something much more, and certainly not something to be ignored.

I think if I had refused Victoria's request, she would have delayed putting on her helmet until the departure time was acceptable. She would have made a scene if she had to, or hid from me if necessary. She knew that we couldn't leave on time, and I believed her without hesitation.

We heard later of a collision that afternoon a few blocks from the route we were taking. I can't be absolutely certain that one of those vehicles would have plowed into our parade of bikes if we had been on schedule. Maybe the changing of our plans completely prevented the accident altogether. Regardless, I mouthed a silent thank-you to my mom when we arrived safely at our destination.

I still do not fully understand the depth of Victoria's gift. I know there are many days that she does not perceive it as a gift. We are often burdened by challenges whose benefits are not realized until years later. It is how we deal with these challenges that make us into stronger people.

Just as the number of crystal children is growing, so is the belief in their abilities. Most people believe in a life after death, so why is hard to believe that people who are "open" can communicate with them? While I am not sure if I would want this gift, I believe it is given for a purpose. It is up to each person how they use what they are given.

For the rest of us, be content in knowing that the loved ones whom we have lost are still with us.

10 - WE MUST CARRY ON

It appears that we have reached the end, or at least the end of this volume. I sincerely hope that I do not have enough future dramatic experiences to warrant another.

Movies of time travel and the ramifications of any alteration to the past have always fascinated me. To be honest, I would be terrified if I had the option to go back and change anything. How overprotective would I have become to try and save my Samantha? Could any change have altered her own short life-path? What alternative future would have my world become if I had chosen the path to the left rather than the right at any of those many forks? Some of those intersections were obviously crucial decisions, such as retreating back to the beach and moving south. Other splits are not even recognized at the time, the diverging pathway overgrown or overlooked as we run past. Only when we look back do we realize that there was another opportunity available.

Regretting the path not taken is a muse to pass the time. The path you have chosen and the future that lies before you is all that matters. Living in the past requires looking backwards. Remembering what is in your rear view mirror, while staying focused on what lies ahead – that will get you to your destination safely.

Remember there is nothing inherently wrong with constructing another addition to your house. There is nothing wrong with settling in and spending your days in the room you are happiest in. The choice is yours. Choices should be weighed and measured carefully, for they often impact others and many hallways in your house are actually one-way streets. Your house is what you make it. Whether you choose to keep the items left behind by visitors is up to you. The hardware stores are always open and your neighbours will lend a hand, if you ask.

Build your community up, for your own house will benefit as well. Helping others adds insulation to your house, keeping you warm and safe from the elements. Remember that the strength of your house will someday form the foundation for your children. They will remember how your house felt and be inclined to fashion their own in that manner.

Keep your board tethered securely. Take every opportunity to make it bigger and easier to find if you slip beneath the surface. There is no shame in asking for a hand up. There is no greater responsibility than to help those who may not have both feet securely planted on their own surfboard.

Depression and despair live in the darkness. Keep your light strong and the sadness cannot flourish. Let down your walls to let others in, for we are strongest when we are together. We are at our best when we love; so love unconditionally and with all your heart. Even if your time together is temporary, the benefits are always worth the risk. If you are lucky, as I have been, you will find yourself in a place that you never thought you would reach.

I cannot overemphasize the word perspective. Things can always be worse and things can always get better. Be grateful for what and who you have, for nothing in life is guaranteed.

Your children are your ultimate second chance. While they have their own free will and determine their own path, the influence you have on them cannot be undervalued. You not only provide the foundation but are crucial to their ground floor. You provide so much of the materials required for construction, and only you affect the integrity and quality of those materials. The most important materials are transferred subconsciously, absorbed through exposure. Empathy and a sense of right and wrong are not taught in classroom, but are ingested gradually from the environment. Keep your environment healthy and good things will grow.

Live your lives as you hope your children will, for they learn by example. Say "I love you" often and more importantly show that love. Hug your children every day, for they are not as indestructible as they should be.

Speak from your soul and empower others with your strength. Overcome your challenges and use them to propel yourself forward. Step on those boulders rather than hide in their shadow or be crushed below them.

The future lies ahead. Today you may find that concept ludicrous. Tomorrow could be darker than today, but there is a light at the end. Sometimes that light will come to us, but more often than not we must continue moving in order to reach it. You can do anything that you set your mind to. The only thing that you cannot do, that you must not do, is give up.

Together we must carry on.

ABOUT THE AUTHOR

Bob currently lives in Southwestern Ontario with his wife, Lori, and two children, Victoria and Noah. The R.O.C.K. continues to roll for childhood cancer research, having raised over $300,000 for Childhood Cancer Research as of 2013. Two fictional books are in the works.

Made in the USA
San Bernardino, CA
10 November 2013